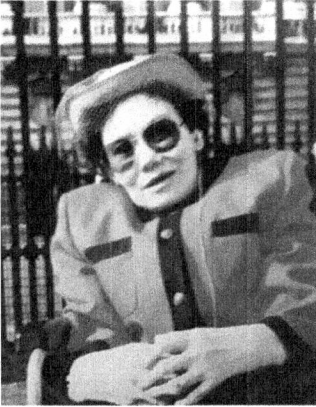

were told that their first child had been born with a rare bone disorder which in turn would mean that she wouldn't survive. How wrong they were. Not only did she survive, but her achievements went far beyond all expectations.

Elisabeth rose to great heights, not least achieving a First Class Honours degree in Philosophy. Along with all her other academic skills she went on to enhance the lives of many, ensuring equality for all disabilities in the workplace (this she achieved in her position as Equalities Officer at Bristol City Council).

Not satisfied with workplace equality, she went on to teach professionals in many fields from universities to hospitals. Her aim was always centred around her personal experiences at the hands of professionals who had little or no knowledge of the individual needs of disabled people.

Elisabeth's hard work was recognised when, in 1992, she was awarded an MBE for her services to disabled people. She went on to chair the Bristol Disability Forum, and the Association of Blind and Partially Sighted Teachers and Students. Her achievements had no bounds, and she thrived on them all. After her retirement she discovered the joy of writing, from short stories to poetry, followed by this memoir (*The Red Coat*).

THE
RED
COAT

A Memoir of Blindness

Elisabeth Standen

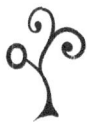

SilverWood

Published in 2024 by SilverWood Books

SilverWood Books Ltd
14 Small Street, Bristol, BS1 1DE, United Kingdom
www.silverwoodbooks.co.uk

ISBN 978-1-80042-273-5 (paperback)

Also available as an ebook

British Library Cataloguing in Publication Data
A CIP catalogue record for this book is
available from the British Library

Page design and typesetting by SilverWood Books

**All proceeds from the sale of copies of this book, once production costs
have been covered, will be donated to Deafblind UK and other disability
charities that Elisabeth supported.**

Contents

Introduction

My sister Elisabeth Florence Carina was born on 16 October 1944, the first child of our parents Philip and Hetty Worton. Shortly after her birth our parents were told that she had been diagnosed with a severe but obscure bone disorder and it was unlikely that she would survive into her teenage years. It soon also became apparent that she was blind in one eye. The consultant recommended that they leave her in the hospital and go home and carry on with their lives as if she had never been born. But in 1914 our father Philip had been born in a workhouse before being brought up in an orphanage. At the age of twelve he had found himself out on the street, having to fend for himself. Now, thirty years later, there was no way Dad was going to abandon his newborn child. Against all advice, our parents insisted on taking Elisabeth home.

They lived in a tied cottage, with no running water and no electricity, on the farm where Dad worked as an agricultural labourer. This was before the days of the NHS, and they had to pay for any medical services Elisabeth needed. Yet she thrived at home with them. When she was two they moved to a place near Oxford with running water but still no electricity; this was where our brother Philip was born, followed by me two years later. Mum was struggling with three small children and Dad once more found himself looking for better employment along with more suitable accommodation, which after some time he found on a farm in Warwickshire. Mum couldn't believe her luck: the cottage had not only running water, but also electricity. For the first few days she was constantly switching the lights on and off, in awe of this miracle. She grew vegetables and kept chickens, and although Elisabeth's medical costs were a constant challenge, we got by.

Just before Elisabeth turned five, she started at the village school. Everyone was amazed by how quickly she fitted in. She soon learned to read and write, and although she was much smaller than the other children it didn't stop her from joining in with their games. But sadly, the local council's education department decided that she was in danger of injury from the other children, and decreed that she be removed from the school. In those days – not so long ago – families had no say in decisions that were made under the guise of them being 'in their best interest'.

Some months later, with Elisabeth at home not understanding why she couldn't play with her school friends any longer, Mum and Dad were told that a place had been found for her at a boarding school a few miles away. Although they were opposed to this decision there was nothing they could do. Being sent to this school was catastrophic for Elisabeth. She had two falls: one, incredibly, out of the door of the school minibus, and the other down a flight of stairs. When she told members of staff that she suddenly couldn't see anything, she was accused of telling lies and was punished. When Mum visited the following weekend she found Elisabeth in the sickbay and realised at once that she had lost her sight. At the eye hospital, to which Elisabeth was finally taken, it was discovered that she had suffered a detached retina in her good eye. She was now totally blind. Had she been taken to hospital, or just to a doctor, at the time of the first accident, her sight could very possibly have been saved.

Elisabeth came home. Every morning our brother Philip would go off cheerfully to primary school – the very one where Elisabeth had been so happy – while she stayed at home with me and Mum. A Braille teacher used to come once a week, but otherwise there was nothing for Elisabeth to do.

A year passed by, and then a letter came from the education department saying that a school for the blind and physically challenged in Shropshire had been found which might be willing to take her. Our parents took her on a visit and the school accepted her. Our parents didn't want her to go; they thought something even worse might happen at this school than had happened at the previous one. But their wishes, their anxieties, and what they thought would be best for their daughter and for the whole family were not taken into account, and off Elisabeth went. Working-class parents were not deemed capable of knowing what was best for their disabled child. That was then. I believe, and sincerely hope, that things are arranged differently now.

Elisabeth stayed at the school in Shropshire until she was fifteen, and although she came back for the holidays it was as if, for my brother and myself during those years, we were a family of four. Once a month the four of us took a train to Shropshire to visit her, and although by now her medical needs were covered by the NHS there was no spare cash, and our monthly visits were funded by Mum going out every day to clean people's houses. Whenever our parents spoke to each other in Welsh – their shared first language – Philip and I knew that there was, if not a crisis, then at least an anxiety that had something to do with Elisabeth. Their worried love for her was the background to our growing up.

In the pages of this book you will encounter the subjective experience of my sister's early years, in which she recounts the trauma of that first boarding school, the hospital stays that sometimes lasted for months, and the way she coped with the hearing loss that followed the loss of her sight. I am not now going to tell you about the rest of Elisabeth's life. She tells it so brilliantly herself. I shall just say that she managed to move herself from a place of despair to heights of remarkable achievement and personal happiness. In her working life she made a huge difference to the lives of many people with disabilities of various kinds. Mum and I were so proud of her the day we went to Buckingham Palace and watched her being awarded an MBE for services to disability. This amazing woman was once the baby whom all the doctors had written off at birth.

I am now going to quote from a memorial piece written by Elisabeth's friend and 'writing buddy', Judy Darley:

> *When she was a small child her parents were told that there were two things she would never do – find love, and survive. She rebelled against both those judgements, and continued to defy expectations throughout her life. Elisabeth was compassionate, determined and endlessly inventive, both in her writing and in the spirited way she approached everyday tasks while challenged by her body. She was a prolific writer, reader and lover of life, surrounded by friends and served by a keen wit coupled with a temper that ensured that anyone who underestimated her (and there were many) soon had their assumptions shaken.*

In this lightly fictionalised memoir, two siblings appear, but they are called Rosemary and Stephen rather than Gwynneth and Philip. The narrator is called Lucy Holland rather than Elisabeth Worton. Lucy meets, falls in love with and marries a man called Harry Ansel; the name of Elisabeth's great love – the man she married – was Charles Standen. Warwick, however, is the university where both Elisabeth and her alter ego Lucy gain their degrees in philosophy, and David Scott Blackhall was indeed the presenter of the BBC's *In Touch*, and an important person in the lives of both Elisabeth and her husband. While Elisabeth was taking her final exams she was also caring for Charles, who was terminally ill, just as Lucy cares for Harry. Elisabeth had a tenacious spirit, which Charles encouraged. His death caused her terrible grief, but she survived it and went on to have a fulfilling career and a rich, independent life. My sister loved playing the piano. She was a keen gardener, and an almost invincible player of Scrabble.

In Bristol in the early 1990s, when Elisabeth was working for the city council as an equalities officer with a specialism in disability, she was contacted by Dennis Casling, a disabled poet who had received a grant to run poetry workshops in the city. 'He rang me up and asked me to go along. I said I didn't do poetry, but Dennis was persistent. He was afraid no one would turn up, so in the end I caved in,' she told Judy Darley in a 2009 magazine interview. 'Those workshops,' wrote Judy, 'were life-changing for Elisabeth.' As Elisabeth said, 'I acquired a compulsion to write poetry!'

At around the same time she attended the first of a series of day schools, run by the access unit at the University of Bristol, on writing memoir and family history. They were taught by Sarah LeFanu, who would become (along with Judy Darley, and others in Elisabeth's writing group) a close critical reader of the memoir/novel that Elisabeth would soon begin to write. *The Red Coat* is the fruit of the work of many years, and of many drafts and revisions. Much of its content – especially, but not only, that concerning Elisabeth's early school years – was very painful for her to recall, and not surprisingly she found it hard to write about. I remember that as a child – the youngest child – I would often say (or shout!), 'It's not fair,' to which Elisabeth would respond, 'Nobody ever told me it was supposed to be fair – so get over it!' And then: 'Nothing is impossible, it's just different – so adapt!'

Not long before her death, Elisabeth was granted a bursary by The Literary Consultancy to have the manuscript of her book read and editorially assessed. This resulted in some profound rethinking. Novel or memoir? Memoir or novel? In my view, it is both.

On 17 June 2020 I found my beautiful, amazing sister lying quietly in her bed at home with her beloved cat Bret beside her. I miss her each and every day, but I believe that her story of dreams and determination, of overcoming huge difficulties, of courage and passion and love, will inspire others as it has inspired me all my life.

Gwynneth Shakespeare, 2024

THE RED COAT

Prologue

My name is Lucy Holland, and one dull July afternoon in 1971, when I was twenty-six years old, I reached a watershed moment in my life. Or perhaps I should say, it was thrust upon me. I was sitting in the front parlour of the Midlands council house where I lived with my parents, knitting a jumper for my sister Rosemary's youngest, and listening to *La Fille Mal Gardée* on the radio, when I heard the doorbell. It had already rung several times that afternoon.

I heard Mum's voice as she let in another visitor. Nothing to do with me. 'The Clog Dance' faded and *Home This Afternoon* was over, but I still hadn't been called to tea and I was beginning to feel hungry. I pushed my needles securely into the ball of wool, put down my knitting, and switched off the radio. I opened the parlour door, and now I heard a babble of voices from the back room. My father's deep voice; my brother Stephen, sounding ill-tempered. What was Stephen doing here? Shouldn't he be at work? And wasn't that Cousin Jill, interrupting Mum? And Jill's husband Dan? Why was all the family here? Was Rosemary here too? I couldn't hear her voice. I hesitated by the door, and heard someone say loudly, 'Shall we tell Lucy?' Surely that was the voice of Miss Briggs, the social worker? What on earth was she doing here?

'No, there's no need to worry Lucy yet.' That was Mum. 'She'll find out soon enough when the time comes for her to go and live with Jill and Dan. No need to worry her just now.'

I opened the door and stepped into the room. My heart was thumping. Blood roared in my ears. 'When am I going to live with Jill and Dan, and why?'

I heard the rattle of teacup and saucer, and then Mum said, 'Not for a long, long time, darling.'

'But why would I go to live with them anyway?' I could hear my voice beginning to rise.

'Well,' said Miss Briggs, in what was probably meant to be a soothing tone, 'at some time in the future – the distant future – your mother and father may not be able to care for you. So we were making plans, just preliminary plans.'

'Don't I have a say in the matter? You're wrapping up my life, and you'll be ordering my coffin next.' I swung around, slammed the door behind me, and stumbled upstairs. Tears gushed from my sightless eyes.

Part One

1

Spring 1949. This must be one of my very first memories. It's Stephen's second birthday, and he has been given a tricycle. I am entranced by the movement; the speed. Look at him go!

'Me, me, let me ride!' I call out from where I'm sitting on the grass.

'No, dear,' says Mummy. 'You won't be able to pedal.'

'Let me! Let me ride.'

'But it's Stephen's bike. It's his birthday.'

Jumping off the trike, Stephen claps his hands and, hopping from foot to foot, chants, 'Lucy ride, Lucy ride, ride, Lucy, Lucy ride.'

I'm two years older than my little brother, but I can't even do that: I can't hop, or walk, or even stand without help.

'Oh, let her have a go,' says Daddy. He scoops me up from the lawn and puts me gently on the saddle, and then places my feet on the pedals. 'Now, try pushing them round.'

I hunch over the handlebars and peer down at my feet. I can't see at all with my right eye, but now that I've got glasses I can see perfectly out of the left one. Slowly I press my weight down on the foot that is highest, and watch the other one come up. Down, up, down, up. The trike jerks forwards. I grip the handlebars. The pedals turn. Slowly, I move down the path, all on my own, with the breeze blowing through my hair.

*

By the summer I've moved on from circling the garden to going out to the lane, up to the bridge, and, in the other direction, down to the road. The humped bridge is gloomy and a little frightening: giants, ogres and wicked witches live on its far side. At the other end of the lane, buses and cars whizz by on the main road. Long grass grows on either side of the rough, bumpy lane; there are dandelion clocks to tell the time, and yellow buttercups that – if you hold them under your chin, Aunty Sally says – will show if you like butter. Red ants drag bits of grass and earth here and there. Sometimes butterflies flutter by, or settle on a flower. This is a new world that Stephen's trike has opened up for me, but I always know that home is just the other side of the dense green hedge.

The lane has its regular visitors, such as old Aunty Jean, who comes huddled up in a long dark coat even on the warmest afternoons, and leans on the bridge, staring into the water. Perhaps the wicked witches have cast a spell over her that makes her sad, for she never smiles. Joe comes sometimes, bringing lumpy sacks of coal for the fire. The dustcart clatters along every Tuesday morning to empty the bins from all four houses in the lane.

Aunty Sally usually arrives at teatime on Thursdays to see Mrs Donaldson at number three. 'Hello, Lucy,' she'll call. 'Want some sticky toffees? Two for you and two for Stephen.' She is pretty in her bright summer dresses and high-heeled sandals.

Uncle Stan from next door often comes home carrying shopping and sometimes a bunch of flowers. Then he'll call out, 'Hey there, Lucy, want a flower?' He'll fasten a daisy or a violet under my hair ribbon, and then I'll pedal home to show Mummy and Stephen.

Best of all, every day at teatime Daddy comes home from his work on the farm a few miles away and turns into the lane on his bike.

'Daddy, Daddy!' I shout, and pedal as fast as I can to meet him.

He lifts me off the trike and wraps me in a bear hug, and I inhale his warm smells of hay and earth and cows. Then he puts me back on the trike and we race each other home.

2

In September, when I'm nearly five, I start at the village school. That first morning, I feel so excited I can hardly breathe. Sunshine streams into the hall through the high windows, lighting up the front bench.

'Good morning, children,' says the headmistress.

'Good morning, Mrs Watson.'

I watch her eagerly.

'We have several new children joining us today,' she says. 'David Markham, Angela Bennet, Malcolm Brown and Lucy Holland. They are all joining Miss Barnes's class. I am sure you older children will be kind and show them around.' She looks directly at me and gives me a big smile.

I smile back.

'Now, children, I have something very serious to say to you all. It is about one of our new pupils, Lucy Holland. Lucy is a little small for her age and has some difficulties walking, so I want you all to be careful not to knock her over. At playtime she will go into the playground with her classmates, but she will probably sit on the steps and watch the games. I am sure some of you will spend some time talking to Lucy and letting her get to know you.' She smiles at me again. 'Now, we'll end this first assembly of the new school year by singing "All Things Bright and Beautiful".'

*

'Jelly on a plate, jelly on a plate. Wibble, wobble, wibble, wobble—'

'It's my turn to skip now,' says a girl with yellow hair.

'OK,' says another. 'Mandy and I will turn the rope.'

I sit on the step, and watch them with longing. How I'd love to do skipping.

'Lucy's watching – do you think she wants to play?' asks one.

'She won't be able to skip,' the one called Mandy points out.

'No, but perhaps she could turn the rope.'

'Let's ask her,' says the first girl. She comes over to where I'm sitting. 'Want to play?'

'I… I can't skip.'

'But couldn't you turn the rope?'

Yes, of course I could.

'I'm Michelle, that's Mandy, and she's Jane.'

And then I'm chanting with them. *'Jelly on a plate, jelly on a plate. Wibble, wobble, wibble, wobble, jelly on a plate.'*

Jane, the one who suggested I could turn the rope, lives down the lane from me, and while the evenings are still light we often play together in the lane after school.

Only a few weeks into term, my ear starts hurting, and it gets worse and worse, like a fire burning deep down inside my ear. When Mummy takes me to the doctor, he sends me on to another doctor at the hospital, and that doctor says I have to stay in the hospital. A nurse comes with a wheelchair and wheels me out of the room and away from Mummy, down a long, noisy corridor full of hurrying people, around a corner and through some double doors, and one of them swings back and hits me on my hand where it's lying on the armrest. I scream out loud, and the nurse is angry. She tells me to shush and not make a noise. When we get to the children's ward I can't raise myself out of the wheelchair:

my wrist where the door slammed into me is red and puffy, and I can't move my hand at all. They take an X-ray the next day: my wrist is fractured.

I stay in hospital for a week or so. When I get home, Jane doesn't come round any more to ask me to play, and at school I have to sit on the step like I did at the beginning of term and watch the others skipping. No one asks me to hold the rope.

'Mummy, they won't play with me any more,' I cry on the way home.

'I'm sorry, darling, but their mummies are afraid that if you play together you might get hurt and they will be blamed.'

'But Jane, Mandy and Michelle don't hurt me.'

'I know, love, but they are afraid. It's silly, but they also think their little girls might end up with wonky bones likes you.'

'That's not fair.'

'I agree, love.' Mummy stoops down and hugs me. 'But nothing I say will change their minds.'

'Why are my bones wonky?'

'They just are.'

But I still love school: I love story time and quiet reading; I love singing and counting; I love painting. The other children are still very friendly with me, even if they don't ask me to play with them. David Markham says I'm really pretty and sometimes tries to kiss me; Mandy, Michelle and Jane let me join in when they're combing each other's hair. They say I've got lovely super-long ringlets, and they love tying ribbons in them. When Stephen starts school, the others are jealous that I've got a little brother I can boss around, even though he's already taller than I am. By then we've got another baby at home: a sister called Rosemary.

*

Then one Saturday, everything changes. Mummy and Daddy, with very serious faces, tell me to come and sit down in the parlour. They tell me that I'm not going back to school, but instead I'm going to a new one. They call it a 'special school'.

'But why?' I cry. 'Will Jane, Michelle and Mandy go too?'

'No, dear,' says Mummy, 'but I'm sure you'll soon make lots of new friends.'

'I don't want new friends.' I put my head in my arms and sob. 'I want Jane, Michelle and Mandy to be my friends.'

The worst is yet to come.

'You will share a bedroom with another little girl,' says Mummy. 'You're bound to get on very well.'

'A *bedroom*?' What on earth is Mummy talking about? 'But I've got my own bedroom here.'

'And it will still be here when you come home,' Daddy says, putting an arm around me and hugging me tight.

In a low voice, Mummy says, 'You'll have to stay at the school for a little while.'

'I'm not to come home?' What? I can't believe it. I stare at Mummy, and then at Daddy, and I shake my head and cry out, louder and louder, 'No, no, no!'

'You'll come home during the holidays,' says Daddy.

I start crying then, and I cry and cry and cry. What can I have done to make them send me away?

3

'Can Baby go too?' I clutch the doll tightly to my side. I am seven years old.

'Of course, darling. Baby will need you to look after her,' says Mummy, looking up from where she's kneeling on the floor, packing a suitcase. Two dark green gymslips, two cardigans, vests, socks, knickers. So many clothes I have to take; Mummy ticks off each garment on a list as she puts it in the case. 'What else would you like to take?'

'My Noddy and Big Ears book,' I say, putting it on top of the clothes, 'and my comics.' I go and get them from the toy cupboard.

'Daddy and I will write you a letter every week and send you your comic,' Mummy promises. She closes the lid of the suitcase and clicks the lock shut.

I feel a bit sick.

We're going by bus to Hinton Grange. We'll have to change three times; it's a long journey. Daddy and Stephen wave us off from the bus stop. Even Rosemary, in Daddy's arms, waves her little hand. My uniform is scratchy and uncomfortable, but I don't say anything. Mummy is very quiet.

After forever we get down from the third bus and walk through some huge gates and start to walk up a long, long drive towards a grey building that squats in front of us. Now Mummy grips my hand so tight that it hurts.

'Mummy!'

'Sorry, darling.' There's a wobble in Mummy's voice.

We are shown into a room where a man introduces himself as Mr Morrison, the headmaster, and introduces a woman with thin lips and grey hair scraped back off her forehead. 'This is Mrs Pryce. Mrs Pryce, this is Lucy Holland and her mother.' Mr Morrison turns to Mummy. 'Mrs Pryce is house mother in Kenilworth House, where Lucy will be.'

Mrs Pryce doesn't smile. Nor does Mummy.

'So, this is Lucy,' says Mrs Pryce. She looks me up and down.

'I think you should take Lucy down to the house and settle her in before tea,' Mr Morrison says. 'Now, Lucy, say goodbye to your mother.'

I hang on tight to Mummy's hand and push myself against her legs, and I hear her say, 'I'd like to see where Lucy's going to sleep, and I want to unpack her things.'

'That's not usual,' says Mrs Pryce. I see her look at the headmaster.

'We find it's best if parents say goodbye here and let the house mother settle the child in,' Mr Morrison says.

But Mummy carries on. 'But I want to see her room and do the unpacking myself.'

'Oh, well,' Mr Morrison says, 'perhaps just this once it won't matter.'

Mrs Pryce opens her mouth to say something. She looks again at the headmaster, and shuts it. Then she looks at us and her lips crack open in a thin smile. 'This way,' she says.

*

For many years to come I shall be quite unable to think about any aspect of Hinton Grange. I try to close my mind to it; to get rid of the images that sometimes pop up when I'm least expecting them, as if they're trying to take me unawares. I was torn from an ordinary, happy life and thrown without warning into a noisy, cold, sharp-edged world in which, when a kind word was dropped my way, I'd gather it up and hoard it against what was to come. I never want to think back to it.

But later, when I'm older, stronger and happier, when Harry has his arms around me and I feel safe, I'll look back, and I'll begin to see what I couldn't see then, when I was only seven. I shall understand that my mother and father only allowed me to go to Hinton Grange because they couldn't do anything else. They were in thrall to the middle-class professionals who decided what was best for their disabled daughter. Who were they, after all? Just a farm labourer and his wife who worked part-time as a cleaner, living in a council house. I shall remember that moment in Mr Morrison's study when my mother stood up to him and Mrs Pryce, and insisted that she see where her daughter was going to be sleeping. Many years later, I shall salute my mother's courage on that day.

Mrs Pryce leads the way to Kenilworth House. The path ends in a small stile. Mrs Pryce lifts me over it. The building is long and low, but not all on one level. Inside the entrance is a large communal area with a corridor leading off it where the toilets are. Some shallow stone steps lead up from the communal area to a narrow corridor with bedrooms off it on either side. I am to share with a girl called Mattie.

Mrs Pryce leaves us alone so that Mummy can help me unpack. 'You've got fifteen minutes before tea,' she says as she goes out.

Mummy chatters as she unpacks my suitcase and puts my things away. All those horrid clothes I have to have. 'It won't be long before I'll be fetching you home for the holidays,' she says brightly.

I sit on the bed, hugging Baby tight. Mummy won't come back, I'm thinking, Mummy won't come back.

At the dining-room door, Mrs Pryce calls out, 'Mattie White?'

A girl runs up. She's got brown hair in two plaits, and she's bigger than me, but not much bigger. 'Yes, Mrs Pryce?'

'This is Lucy. She's going to be sharing your room.'

Mattie smiles at me. I creep closer to Mummy.

'Now,' says Mrs Pryce briskly, 'say goodbye to your mother, Lucy, and go off to tea with Mattie.'

Mummy bends and hugs me and gives me a kiss. She whispers, 'Be good for Mummy. I'll come to fetch you very, very soon.' Then she turns and walks quickly towards the gate. At the last minute she turns and waves.

I raise my arm. What if I never see Mummy, or Daddy, or Stephen or Rosemary ever again? As I turn away, I hear the gate clang shut.

That night, I huddle up under the blankets and try to stifle my sobs. One, two, three buses. I count on my fingers. What if Mummy gets lost on the buses and can't come back to get me? A wave of sobbing shakes my whole body. I want to go home, I want to go home…

4

I wake up to the clanging of a bell.

'Time to get up,' says Mattie, and she jumps out of bed.

I do the same. A rising tide of chatter sweeps in from the corridor outside.

Mrs Pryce appears in the doorway. 'Good, Lucy. I see you're up. Get dressed quickly and bring me your brush and I'll do your hair.'

I follow Mattie; hairbrush in one hand and Baby tucked under the other arm.

'Here, these are your sandals, Lucy. You should really have shoes at this time of year. Put them on, then I'll brush your hair,' says Mrs Pryce. 'Ringlets are all very pretty, I'm sure, but they're so much trouble. And what are you doing with that doll?'

'I'm carrying her. Baby can't walk, Mrs Pryce.'

'Go and put her on your bed. You're a big girl now. Big girls don't take their dolls to breakfast.'

I go back to the bedroom and put Baby carefully on the pillow. 'I'll be back very soon, Baby,' I promise her.

Then I hear a raised voice. 'Come on, Lucy. We haven't got all day.'

A group of girls are standing in a line in the hallway, their hands held out towards the looming figure of Mrs Pryce. I join Mattie at the end of the line.

'Show me your nails, Lucy,' orders Mrs Pryce. 'Yes, they'll do.' She walks to the front of the line, says, 'Quick march,' and off we go behind her, two by two, out of the door and towards the main block and breakfast.

They all walk incredibly fast. I'm having to run to keep up. But I can't. I'm stumbling.

'Mrs Pryce, Mrs Pryce!' one of the girls calls out. 'Lucy's being left behind.'

Mrs Pryce stops, and everyone turns around. She calls out crossly, 'Mattie, you and Lucy had better come up here where I can keep an eye on you both.'

I limp up to the head of the line as fast as I can, past all the other girls, my legs aching.

We all sit around a table at one end of a large dining room. Bigger girls and boys are sitting at the other tables. It is very noisy. Mrs Pryce dishes out a bowl of porridge for each of us and pours out tea. A glass container with a shiny chimney on top is passed from hand to hand, and everyone tips it up over their porridge. Ah. It's sugar. Not much comes out, but I don't think we're allowed to tip it twice. A bell rings and everyone jumps up, scraping their chairs as they push them under the table. Someone sings a short grace.

'Lucy, you go with Miss Williams,' says Mrs Pryce to me once we've filed out of the dining room. Then she turns and walks off with the other girls.

A fair-haired woman is smiling down at me. 'Come with me, Lucy,' she says. 'We're going this way. Can you manage steps?'

I nod, and reach for the handrail. At the bottom of the stairs we turn right and go through a door, where a small group of girls, some big and some small, are clustered around a sink, brushing their teeth.

'Eileen,' says Miss Williams, 'this is Lucy Holland. Give her a toothbrush, please.'

Eileen is one of the older-looking girls, and she walks with crutches.

'When you've all finished, show her the way to the assembly hall,' continues Miss Williams. 'Quick, now – we're running late.'

Assembly follows. We sing some hymns, listen to a reading by Eileen that I don't really understand (something to do with wheat and tares), and then there's a talk by Mr Morrison (also about tares – or is it perhaps tears?). Then we sing another hymn, and then names are called out and children get up and go and stand in line.

'Lucy Holland,' I hear, and someone pushes me to my feet and directs me to one of the groups. Mattie is already there – phew, that's a relief, and even better, there's Miss Williams again, smiling and clucking at us and leading us out of the hall.

The classroom seems to be miles away, but we get there at last.

'Here, Lucy, you can sit next to Mattie. We have reading first. Can you read?'

'Yes, Miss Williams.' Of course I can read!

At break time we line up and take a straw from a box on Miss Williams's desk, and then pick up a small bottle of milk from a crate that's been left outside the door. In the playground I sit with Mattie and suck up my milk. After break we do sums until dinner time. I like doing sums. When the dinner bell goes, Miss Williams tells us to close our books and get our coats. She tells me to go with her, and explains that some of the handicapped children get a ride to dinner. It's a high step up into the van – too high for me to manage. Miss Williams picks me up and lifts me in, and tells me to go and sit on the back seat next to Eileen, the big girl with crutches who did the reading at assembly. After dinner we all have to play outside in the field, then it's back to the classroom until tea, and then we go back to our separate houses.

And so time passes. Every day is the same: breakfast, assembly, lessons, dinner, play, lessons, tea and then bed. Before bed we line up for a spoonful of malt and cod liver oil. Then we have to take off our shoes and put them neatly on a platform near the top of the steps at the end of the corridor, along with our hair ribbons. I don't know why. I always seem to be struggling to get to the next place on time. During the day there's not a spare second to think of home, but at night, in bed at last, I feel a wave of homesickness sweeping over me. Every night I curl up beneath the blankets, holding Baby tight, and the tears flow out of me until at last I fall into the darkness of sleep. Sometimes I wake up in the middle of the night needing a wee, but it's very dark down the steps to the toilet corridor and I'm too scared to try. I have to hold it in until morning comes. But one night I don't manage it, and when I wake up the bed is wet.

That evening, Mrs Pryce is waiting for me. 'You're a dirty girl, Lucy Holland,' she shouts as I come in the front door.

Everybody turns and stares at me. I feel my face turn hot and I want the ground to swallow me up.

'Wetting the bed at your age. It's disgusting. Well, you'll have to sleep alone tonight.'

After the malt and cod liver oil, Mrs Pryce takes my arm and drags me to an empty room at the far end of the corridor. 'This is where you'll sleep tonight, Lucy Holland. You're a very wicked, dirty girl. You know what happens to wicked girls, don't you? Something nasty comes through the door from outside, and takes them away in the middle of the night. And dirty girls can't have their dolls to sleep with them, either.' She turns off the light, bangs the door shut, and leaves me all alone in the dark.

All night I lie awake, my eyes straining towards the door. I'm frightened, Mummy. Please come and take me home. But Mummy doesn't come.

5

The worst thing about the path between Kenilworth House and the main school building is the stile. It's not very high, but it's awkward and I just can't manage it. For the first few days Mrs Pryce lifts me over it, but one evening as we're going back to the house after tea she refuses to, saying, 'I'm sure you could manage it if you tried.' She watches me as I struggle and struggle; then she just picks me up and dumps me roughly on the other side.

The next day, Mrs Pryce isn't there, so I sit on the black water pipe that's next to the stile and swing my legs across, which isn't that difficult. But the following morning, Mrs Pryce spots some telltale black marks on the back of my gymslip.

'I don't know what we're going to do with you,' she says coldly.

A few days later I find that the pipe has been covered in barbed wire. I have to be very, very careful. What she'll do to me if I tear my clothes just doesn't bear thinking about.

Saturday is tuck shop day. After breakfast, we get given our weekly sixpence, and set off for the assembly hall. The first week I stick close to Mattie as we join the queue of children snaking around the room. When we reach the front, Mattie climbs the two steps up to the stage, but they're awfully high, and I'm not sure I can manage them. Suddenly I am picked up, whirled through the air, and put down gently next to Mattie. A tall, fair-haired boy with thick glasses is grinning down at me.

'There you go,' he says, laughing.

'Thank you,' I whisper, looking down at my feet.

On one side of the stage, two smiling women sit behind a table with shelves ranged behind them.

'Well, here's a new little girl. What's your name, dearie?' one of them asks.

'Lucy. Lucy Holland,' I whisper.

'Well, Lucy Lucy Holland, what are you going to spend your sixpence on?'

I look at all the glass jars on the shelves. Everything is there: dolly mixtures; jelly babies; humbugs; pear drops; sugared almonds; sherbet lemons; tubes of wine gums, Spangles and Polos; Toffee Cups wrapped in shiny paper; triangular Sherbet Fountains with their liquorice sticks; Liquorice Allsorts; and Maltesers. How on earth can I choose?

'Well, dearie, what's it to be?'

I ask for a Sherbet Fountain and a Toffee Cup, and hand over my sixpence. Then I turn to go.

'There you are!' It's the tall boy again. He picks me up once more and swings me down off the stage. 'What do I get now?' he asks gruffly.

I don't look at him, but hold out my sweets and try not to cry.

'That's OK, poppet, you keep them,' he says, and pats me on the head. 'I'm only teasing. My name's Alec, by the way. What's yours?'

6

Mummy doesn't get lost: she gets on the three different buses and finds her way back to the school to pick me up, so I do go home for the holidays. But all too soon the holidays are over, and then it is three long bus rides back to Hinton Grange.

Another term goes by. I seem to find it more and more difficult to manage stairs, or rough ground. Even walking in the corridors seems harder. The footpath is a twice-daily nightmare.

I am examined by the school doctor, and he says I have to go to a specialist at the hospital in Coventry. I don't mind: it means being away from Hinton Grange, and being with Mummy.

I lie under a blanket in a curtained cubicle, wearing only my knickers. The curtain opens and a man in a white coat comes in, with lots of other white-coated men pressing in behind him. The one in front introduces himself to Mummy as Mr Ryder.

'You don't mind students, do you?' Without waiting for her to reply, he turns to look at me lying on the trolley and says briskly, 'Achondroplasia. Cause unknown. Probably genetic mutation.' He takes the blanket off me. 'Note the outsized knee joints and ankles.' He bends my right leg, straightens it, takes my foot in his huge hand and flexes the ankle joint. 'Note the limited movement,' he says to his students. He does the same with my left leg. Then he pulls the blanket back up to my chest and picks up my arms, one after the other, bending the elbows. 'Note that she cannot reach her shoulders. Now, make a fist for me.'

I clench my fingers together as tight as I can.

'See, they can't hold things properly – it's more like clawing at them. Now, show us how you walk.' He scoops me up from the trolley and lowers me onto my bare feet on the faded carpet. 'See if you can follow that white line.'

My legs feel weaker than usual – I think because I've been lying on the trolley for so long – and I'm cold without any clothes on except my knickers, but I struggle forwards, trying desperately hard to place my feet on the white strip stitched along the carpet. I have to lean forwards, and push my arms out to the sides for balance. 'Left foot, right foot,' I whisper under my breath.

'Good girl,' Mr Ryder says to me kindly. Then he turns to his students. 'You see, she walks on the outside edges of her feet, with her knees bowed out.' Lowering his voice, but not so low I don't hear, he adds, 'Waddling like a drunken duck.'

One of the students gives a guffaw, which he turns into a cough when Mr Ryder glares at him.

'That's enough for today.' Mr Ryder picks me up, lays me back on the trolley and covers me again with the blanket. Then he turns to Mummy. 'Why didn't you take her to a doctor before this?'

'We did.' Mummy's voice wobbles. 'We took her to hospitals in Cardiff and Birmingham, but it was no good. They just took our money and said there was nothing they could do.'

'I see. Well, I think I can help. It will mean operating on both legs. She'll be in hospital for several months, but I think I can get her legs straightened out so that she walks on the flat of her feet instead of on the edges, as she does now. Would you and your husband agree to this?'

'We'll try anything if you think it would help.'

*

I don't see Mr Ryder again until the autumn. It's October, and I am back in the Coventry hospital. Once again I am lying on a trolley. I don't know where Mummy is, and Mr Ryder is looming over me like a troll or a giant, but when he speaks his voice is gentle.

'Hello, Lucy. We're going to give you a little prick so that you go to sleep. When you wake up it will all be over.'

I open my eyes to darkness. I try to move, but my legs are so heavy, as if they are tied down with logs or bricks.

'Is it night?' I feel panic rising within me. 'Where am I?' Whose croaky voice is that?

'Awake at last, are we?' A glimmer of light, and a woman's voice. It's not Mummy.

'Where am I?'

'You're in a side ward after your operation.'

My throat is burning. 'Drink,' I croak.

The nurse holds a feeding cup to my mouth and a trickle of water slips between my lips. I take a gulp, and at once I'm retching.

'Ah-yuck, ah-yuck.'

'All right, pet, it'll be all right.' The nurse places a metal bowl under my chin and gently turns my face to the side.

'Ah-yuck, ah-yuck.' Fat tears course down my cheeks. 'Mummy, Mummy, I want my mummy.'

'I know, pet, but it's the middle of the night and Mummy will be fast asleep.' The nurse wipes my face with a damp flannel. 'You go back to sleep now, and when you wake up, you'll feel a lot better and Mummy will come and see you in the afternoon.'

7

The hospital has its own special routine, and soon I am a part of it. I wake each morning to the sound of the bedpan trolley jangling and banging into the ward. Next comes the washing and teeth-cleaning ceremony. At first it seems strange doing everything in bed, but soon it feels normal. Breakfast next, and then the beds are pushed out onto the terrace, and lessons begin. Reading, writing, sums, geography and history are links in the chain of our days. We are all at school, but at this school we all stay in bed. The routine makes me feel safe. Visiting hours are on Sunday afternoons, outside on the terrace around our beds. Mummy comes every week, and Daddy comes too if they are able to leave Stephen and Rosemary with Aunt Renée and Uncle Bill, or with Cousin Jill.

At the end of November, Miss Heggetty, the senior teacher, starts organising a nativity play that, she says, we can perform for our families when they visit on Boxing Day. When I tell Miss Heggetty that I want to be a fairy, she says there are no fairies in the nativity play, but I can be an angel instead. I don't want to be an angel. I want to be a fairy with a wand that makes magic.

On the Sunday before Christmas the ground is covered with a thin icing of snow. Although we have our lessons indoors now, we're still pushed out onto the terrace on Sundays. We're all hunched beneath mounds of blankets and waterproof covers, and our visitors are bundled up in thick coats, scarves and hats. Mummy and Daddy are here, one on either side of me, their hands holding mine underneath the covers.

There is something that has been worrying me for a while. 'Daddy, do you think Father Christmas will know where to bring my stocking this year?'

Daddy suggests I write Father Christmas a letter, and he'll pop it in a postbox on the way home. I have to ask one of the nurses for a bit of paper and a pencil, and then, still huddled beneath the blankets, I write out my address, 'Central Hospital, Coventry', and then fold my letter carefully in two, write 'Father Christmas, North Pole' on the outside, and give it to Daddy to post.

When I wake up on Christmas morning, the first thing I see is a bulging stocking lying across the bottom of my bed. So Father Christmas did get my letter! I pull out sweets and toys, and in the toe of the stocking I find an orange and a shiny new penny. After breakfast – boiled eggs with soldiers – we open our presents from home. I get a new dress and bonnet for Baby, a book of hymns with a lovely picture on each page, a frilly pink jacket to wear in bed, a deep red velvet hair ribbon, and more sweets. Mr Ryder comes in to see us at the end of dinner, and he sets fire to the Christmas pudding, which Miss Heggetty carries around the ward.

Later, as I'm leafing through my new hymn book, I stop at a picture of some angels dressed as carol singers standing on a doorstep with a lantern. The picture shows the inside of the house as well: children playing with toys in front of a Christmas tree, a mummy and daddy giving out presents, a granny and grandad sitting in front of a fire, a cat asleep on the back of a chair. I wonder what they're all doing at home. I blink away the tears in my eyes.

8

One afternoon in early January, just as Miss Heggetty is handing out our exercise books for an arithmetic class, a woman carrying a large bag comes into the ward and walks straight over to my bed. She says her name is Mrs Hopkins, and she's a physiotherapist.

'You and me are going to go for a walk,' she says.

'We can't,' I tell her. 'It's time for arithmetic.'

I'm amazed when Miss Heggetty interrupts with 'I think we'll let you off this once', and picks up my exercise book and moves on towards Becky in the next bed.

'First of all, we need to find you some boots,' says Mrs Hopkins, opening her bag. 'Let's try this pair. No, they're too big. What about these? Yes, I think they'll do.' She fits them over my plastered feet and laces them up tight. 'Now, put your arms in this dressing gown and we'll stand you up.' She puts her hands under my arms and slides me down the side of the bed until my feet are on the floor. 'There – now you're standing on your own two feet.'

I clutch at the edge of the bed, and gasp for air. 'Dizzy,' I tell her.

'That's all right, pet. Just take a few deep breaths and it will soon pass.'

But panic rises. My head swims. 'Help!' I cry out. 'I'm falling, falling!'

'It'll be fine. Nobody's going to let you fall,' says Mrs Hopkins. 'Now, let's take a few steps. Left foot forward. Now the right foot. Good girl – you're doing fine. That's the way.'

And now, somehow, I'm standing beside Becky's bed. Looking around, I see Miss Heggetty and Mrs Hopkins, and two of the nurses at the far end of the ward, and I remember something I'd forgotten in all the time that I've been in hospital: that everyone else is much taller than me. Somehow, high up on the bed, I seem the same as everybody else, but now it's like it always was: they're much bigger than I am. I feel so small.

Then, 'Wow, look, everyone – Lucy's walking!' That's Becky, from her bed.

The others start clapping. For a moment I forget to be scared, and how small I feel.

'Let's go back to your bed now,' says Mrs Hopkins. 'Good – that's enough for today. We'll have another little walk tomorrow.'

A new link is forged in the chain of my days. Each afternoon, for twenty minutes before lessons begin, Mrs Hopkins and I go for a short walk. By Friday I have stepped down the length of the ward, albeit holding on tightly to Mrs Hopkins's hands.

On Monday she brings in a pair of tripods. I stand by the side of my bed with one in each hand.

'Now I've got eight legs,' I say to Mrs Hopkins.

'Yes,' she says. 'And you can't possibly fall over with that many legs to hold you up.'

I lean on them. It feels strange, but safe.

'Now try picking one up, and move it a little forward. That's right. Now the other one. Now move one leg forward. Now the other one. Good girl, that's the way.'

Soon I can walk down the ward on my own. When Mummy comes on Sunday I walk to the ward door to meet her. I see her in the corridor, talking to Becky's dad, and I call out, 'Mummy, Mummy! Look, look – I'm walking all by myself!'

Mummy turns, and her face seems to crumple up. She runs to me and kneels down beside me to give me a hug. 'Oh, Lucy,' she sobs, 'what a clever, clever girl.'

'But why are you crying? Aren't you pleased?'

'Very, very pleased, darling. Just you wait until I tell Daddy, Stephen and Rosemary.'

The following week, on Wednesday, Mr Ryder comes into the ward after dinner. He stands halfway down the ward, between the two rows of beds, then turns to me and says, 'Do you think you can walk over to me?' He holds out his hand.

I take a deep breath, pick up one of my sticks, and step forwards. One, two, three, four steps and I've done it!

'Good girl.' He pats me on the head. Then he digs in his pocket and pulls out a Toffee Cup.

'For me?'

'For you. Next week we'll have an X-ray, and if everything's all right we'll have those plasters off. How about that?'

It's scary, watching the saw working its way up the plaster. The teeth break through, and I feel a tickling sensation as the saw comes into contact with the cotton wool that's wrapped around my legs.

'That's one leg done. Now let's do the other one,' says the ward sister.

Suddenly, there they are: two prickly, skinny white legs that don't seem to belong to me. A deep red scar runs down each one. I put out my finger and touch one of them. It's shiny and smooth.

'They'll fade in time,' the sister says. 'Now we'll make you some splints.'

The next day, I have my first proper bath in months. It's lovely. The water washes away the prickly look, and my legs look so...straight. Are these really my legs? And now I have to exercise every day, and not just by walking: under Mrs Hopkins's instruction, I have to lift my legs, bend them, and move them forwards, backwards and to the sides.

One afternoon, a man arrives on the ward carrying several boxes. 'Now, young lady,' he says, smiling at me, 'let's choose some shoes for you. Proper shoes this time, not sandals. First, we need to measure your feet.'

All evening I keep looking at the shiny black shoes on the top of my locker. My first proper shoes. I can hardly wait for Mrs Hopkins to come tomorrow. If I'm going to learn to walk in proper shoes, they might let me go home soon. Excitement churns in my stomach, and something else too: fear.

9

'Hey, Lucy Locket, so you're back again.'

I look around, and there's Alec smiling down at me.

'Where have you been, skiving off school for two whole terms?'

I tell him that I've been in hospital.

'Looks like you've been on the rack, if you ask me. I swear you've grown. Keep this up and we won't have a school fairy any more.' He ruffles my hair before running off to join his mates.

It's around about now that I begin to visualise my life as if it's happening in two separate boxes. Some of the time I live in the nice home box with Mummy, Daddy, Stephen and Rosemary. Then, just as my memories of school are fading, I am dumped back into the school box. The different boxes are far apart; somehow it always seems a lot further than three bus rides.

The school box is dark, with only chinks of light bringing news from home. I learn to block out my memories of home; thinking about it makes me too sad. I push myself back into the routine of lessons and playtime, of malt and cod liver oil before bed, of waking in the middle of the night and trying desperately not to think about needing to go to the toilet, of being crammed into the van that takes the handicapped children to the main building for dinner and tea. I hate the van. I hate the noise of everyone chattering at once, and I hate having to stand between the front passenger seat and the door, which us smaller girls take it in turns to do. The van is too crammed for everyone to get a seat.

When I'm in the home box I try as hard as I can not to think about that other, darker box that is waiting to enclose me.

The summer and autumn terms pass and it's Christmas again. For Christmas there is another box – of quite a different kind. It's from Cousin Jill: a heavy parcel wrapped in shiny red paper with sprigs of holly on it. Inside is a wooden box. I lift the lid.

'Oh, how pretty! A lady and gentleman – they look as though they're dancing.'

'Look, Lucy,' says Stephen. 'There's a key on the bottom.'

'It's a musical box,' says Daddy. 'Wind it up and let's hear the tune.'

The key is quite stiff but I manage it, and put the box carefully on the floor. 'The Blue Danube' begins to play, and the two figures waltz around the floor of their miniature ballroom.

'Oh, it's beautiful. So very, very beautiful.'

In the years ahead, whenever I hear 'The Blue Danube', I will be transported back to that cosy parlour, with its warm fire and the Christmas tree, and I'll see myself sitting on the floor between my little brother and sister, with the musical box beside me. The image will always shine clear in my mind; a bright picture of warmth and happiness standing out from the encroaching shadows.

10

Back inside the school box in January, I wake early one morning. Oh no! I am desperate for a wee, but I don't want to go down the creepy corridor to the toilet. But I don't want to sleep in the punishment room, either. Perhaps, if I lie very still, I can wait till getting-up time. But that's not going to work, and I scramble out of bed and into my dressing gown and slippers, then grab my glasses and dash down the dimly lit corridor. Perhaps it won't be too late.

At the very top of the stone stairs, my foot meets air instead of the solid step. I'm flying – or am I falling? And then I hear someone screaming. I think it might be me.

'Lucy Holland, what are you doing out of bed at this time?' hisses a voice. 'Stop that noise at once – you'll wake everybody up.'

I am picked up roughly from the floor and shaken hard.

'Oh, not again! You've wet your nightie, and your glasses are broken. I'll have to put you in the bath. What a troublesome child you are.'

'Why are you limping, Lucy?' asks Mrs Parker, as I approach her desk to collect a milk straw.

I'm scared of my new form teacher; the boys call her 'Barker Parker'. 'My leg hurts, Mrs Parker.'

She barks now: 'And where are your glasses?'

'I… I broke them falling downstairs.'

'Well, you and Mattie had better stay in here to drink your milk. It's cold out there and you can't run around to keep warm with a leg like that,' she says, to my surprise. 'And later on, I think you should go and see the physio.'

I go to see the school physiotherapist after dinner.

'Let's have a look at that leg,' Mrs Thomas says. She picks me up and lays me on the couch. 'Hmm, you seem to have sprained it. How did you come to fall downstairs, anyway?'

'Going to the toilet in the dark,' I tell her. And then I admit, in a whisper, 'I'm afraid of the dark.'

'Well, I think a little session under the sun lamp will help to ease it.'

As I lie with my legs warming in the tunnel, I let myself, bit by bit, go soft and limp.

'Here, you can look at the pictures in this book.'

It always feels safe and warm here in Mrs Thomas's room. I wish I could stay here. Of course, I can't stay here forever, but I'm allowed to come every afternoon this week. Mrs Pryce says nothing about sleeping in the punishment room, so that's a relief, and for the rest of the week I spend each afternoon with Mrs Thomas and the sun lamp, looking at picture books, resting, and sometimes chatting when Mrs Thomas isn't busy doing something else.

On Friday she gives me a Babar the Elephant book. I'm looking at a page where Zephir the monkey is being pulled out of a big bowl of custard he's fallen into, when suddenly the picture goes fuzzy round the edges. I blink and it clears. I turn the pages – Zephir is playing the violin and Arthur the cello, in front of

King Babar and Queen Celeste – it happens again. Fuzziness; shadows at the edges of the page.

A few days later I stumble over the milk crate outside the classroom door, fall down, and bang my head on the concrete floor.

'Paul Bennett,' barks Mrs Parker, 'I saw you push Lucy. Now you'll have to stay in and write a hundred lines: "I must not push little girls over."'

But I don't think I was pushed. Paul Bennett is quite rough, but I'm sure it wasn't him.

I hear him whining, 'But, Mrs Parker…' as Mrs Parker helps me up.

'Stop that crying, Lucy, there's no need to make such a fuss,' she says. 'Here's your milk. Now go out and drink it with Mattie. You need some fresh air to put colour back in your cheeks – you're much too pale these days.'

In the van to the dining hall, Eileen is complaining of the crush. This term it's worse than it has ever been. 'They should do two runs instead of cramming us all in like this,' I hear her grumbling from her seat at the back.

It's my turn to stand – again. Mrs Joyce climbs into the driving seat, and the van sets off with a jerk. I try to cling on to the seat beside me, but the big boy sitting there shoves me away. The van swings sharply around a corner, and all at once I'm no longer on my feet. I'm flying backwards. There's a rush of air in my ears, then silence and darkness.

Vaguely, I hear a voice I think I know; a boy's voice. 'Lucy Locket, what are you doing there? Lucy Locket, talk to me. Please talk to me.' Is that somebody holding my hand? Then silence again.

The next thing I know, my face is being sprinkled with water; cold water that seeps under my collar and down my neck.

'Come on, Lucy, wake up. Come on, wake up.' This is a different, louder voice.

I open my eyes. There's a hammer inside my head.

'Come on, Lucy, you've just had a fall.' It's Mrs Parker. 'No need to cry like that. And here's Mrs Joyce, come to find you.'

'Is she all right?' Mrs Joyce is whispering.

They bundle me into the front of the van, where I sit on Mrs Parker's lap. Mrs Joyce jumps back behind the wheel and starts the engine. The two of them bicker over my head – something about a door not being locked, and swinging open.

'We needn't say anything about the van,' says Mrs Parker firmly, 'just that Lucy has had a fall.'

At the sickbay, they hand me over to Nurse Richardson.

I spend a couple of nights in the sickbay, and the hammer in my head eases up. But when I come out, everything looks sort of misty and far away. It's difficult to work out exactly where things are. I keep bumping up against walls, doors and furniture, and knocking things over. Mrs Parker whacks me across the legs with a cane if I bump into something in the classroom.

'Careful, dearie,' says the cleaner one morning after I trip over her bucket in the corridor, slopping the water everywhere.

'Sorry, sorry.' I shrink against the wall and try to disappear.

'Never mind, dearie. No bones broken. Here, have a peppermint.' The woman puts it in my hand and closes my fingers around it. 'How's your dolly? I saw her snuggled up in your bed when I was cleaning your room the other day. What's her name?'

'Baby,' I tell her.

'Baby, that's nice. Well, I'd better get on before the Dragon Pryce catches me slacking.'

'Hey, Lucy Locket, why are you walking past and ignoring me? I thought we were friends.'

I spin around. 'Oh, Alec, I didn't see you.'

'Well, I'm glad you're about again. You gave me a fright, you know.'

I smile at him vaguely. I have no idea what he's talking about, and of course I can't ask him.

Snow falls. It makes it even harder for me to judge the edges of paths, where steps start and stop, and where grass turns to gravel.

'Come on, Lucy,' Mrs Parker says one morning. 'Do you intend to turn up for class today or not?'

'It's difficult to find my way in the snow,' I tell her. 'I can't really see properly.'

'Now, let's have no more of this nonsense. You know perfectly well that when you last saw Dr Shorland he said there was nothing whatsoever wrong with your eye.'

'Sorry, Mrs Parker.'

'Well, now you're here, get on with writing your letter home.'

When it's my turn to take my letter up to the front for inspection, I catch my foot on something – I think it's the leg of a desk in the front row – and I lurch forwards, only just managing not to fall.

'Really, Lucy, you are clumsy these days,' says Mrs Parker, sighing. 'Can't you look where you're going, child?' She snatches the sheet of paper out of my hand. 'What on earth is this?' She's really barking now. 'Your handwriting is all over the place. I won't accept such sloppy work.'

'I can't see the paper properly,' I whisper, cringing away from her loudness.

'Now, I told you what would happen if you made that excuse again. Hold out your hand.'

I hold it out, palm down. It's the only way I can hold it.

'Turn it over.'

'But I can't, Mrs Parker.'

Mrs Parker barks, 'Well, I'll have to hit you on the knuckles, then.'

She strikes my knuckles three times with the ruler. It is agonising.

11

The following week, I'm back in the sickbay. I've just discovered that there will be no going home at half-term: the snow is still falling and roads are closed, bus routes cancelled, and trains unable to move because of snow on the line. I hug Baby to me. Everything is dim and misty; maybe the electricity has been weakened by the snow, or maybe it's because I can hardly stop crying.

Nurse Richardson comes in. 'Look who's here, Lucy!'

I peer towards the door. I see nothing but shadows.

Then suddenly, 'It's Mummy, darling.' And Mummy, a bit fuzzy round the edges, sits on the bed and scoops me up into a big hug.

I cry and cry and hang on to her tight.

'Now, Lucy, darling, let's see what I've brought you. Here are your two favourite chocolate bars.' She tips something onto the blanket.

I pick them up, one in each hand. 'Thank you, Mummy.' I know the milk chocolate one should have a red wrapper, and the white chocolate one a white wrapper. But to me they both look grey. 'Which one is which?'

'What do you mean?'

I think I've upset her. 'Nothing, Mummy. I'm sorry.'

When Mummy speaks again her voice is different; sort of hesitant and anxious. 'How long have you been in the sickbay?'

'Since Friday last week.'

I feel the mattress tremble as Mummy jumps up. 'Mummy's got to go and see someone, darling. I'll be back very soon.'

She does come back soon and she stays quite a long time, but it seems to me that her mind is elsewhere. When she goes, she promises again that she'll come back soon. But when?

I leave the sickbay and everything goes on as usual. But it's not really as usual. It's so misty all the time, but they say there's nothing wrong with me. Am I imagining it? Why is it so misty? Every night before I go to sleep I pray that when I wake up the next day the mist will have cleared and everything will be as it was. There's no point in saying anything more about it. Nobody believes me.

One morning after breakfast, I've just finished cleaning my teeth when Mrs Joyce bustles into the cloakroom.

'Oh, there you are, Lucy. You're coming for a ride with me. Quick, quick,' she says. 'We mustn't be late. Here, put this on.' She bundles me into a coat, and buttons it up before I have time to tell her it's not my coat.

In the van, she lights a cigarette.

I hold on to the sides of the seat with both hands, and ask, 'Where are we going?'

She takes a big drag on her cigarette. 'You'll find out when we get there,' she says as she exhales.

12

'Here we are,' says Mrs Joyce, turning off the engine and opening her door.

'Where are we?' I ask as she lifts me down.

'We're in Warwick, and you're going to see your mummy.'

'Is Mummy here, then?'

'When we get inside, you'll see.'

'Lucy!' Mummy's voice, and Mummy's arms around me. Then, 'But what's this you've got on? This isn't your coat. It doesn't even fit you.'

'Sorry, Mummy,' I murmur, clinging to her neck.

'Oh dear,' says Mrs Joyce. 'That's my fault, I'm afraid. I was so worried that we might be late that I didn't look properly. Just grabbed the nearest coat and ran.'

Mummy says nothing; she just hugs me harder.

Almost at once, we are called in to see the doctor. It's Dr Shorland, who gives eye tests to all the children at school. He sounds impatient.

'I don't know why you requested this,' he snaps at Mummy. 'There was no change in Lucy's eyesight when I last examined her. But Mr Morrison told me you need reassurance, so this is just an ordinary examination to show you that there's nothing wrong.' He turns to me. 'Now, Lucy, tell me what letter this is on the card I'm holding.'

I can't see a card, let alone a letter. 'Where is it?' I ask.

Dr Shorland makes a tutting sound. 'Are you telling me your daughter can't see this great big card?' He sounds incredulous.

Mummy says firmly, 'My daughter is telling you that. Are you saying you don't believe her?'

Dr Shorland makes a noise like 'Hmph!' and I hear him slap the card down on his desk. 'We'll settle this once and for all. I'll do the atropine test. Look up, Lucy, I'm going to put some drops in your eye.'

I can't help saying, 'Ow!' It really stings.

We have to wait for an hour for the drops to take effect. I sit on Mummy's lap in the waiting room, and I think I probably doze off. Then a nurse comes to take us back into the consulting room. I lie on the couch, and Dr Shorland tells me to look up, look to the left, and look to the right.

Then he gasps, and mutters under his breath, 'Oh my God, oh my God.'

'What?' says Mummy. 'What is it?'

'I'm sorry to have to tell you this, Mrs Holland,' he begins brusquely, 'but as far as I can tell, Lucy has gone completely blind.'

'Blind?' says Mummy faintly.

Blind? I think.

'She needs an emergency operation if we're going to save – or try to save – any of her remaining sight at all. I'm calling for an ambulance to take her to Birmingham where I'll be able to operate.'

'No,' says Mummy. 'Lucy is not going anywhere connected with you.' I have never heard Mummy speak like this to anyone. 'I'm taking her back to the eye specialist who looked after her before she came to Hinton Grange.'

'And where does he practise?'

'Cardiff eye hospital.'

'But I can't get the ambulance to take her there. It's out of our area.'

'I'll get her there somehow.'

'But she has to be kept completely flat with as little movement to her head as possible.'

'I'll take care of that,' says Mummy, as if she has been speaking with authority all her life. 'But I need a note from you to give to the specialist.'

'If you know him as well as you say, you don't need a note.'

'I don't need it,' says Mummy. 'But it would be a courtesy, and I'm not leaving this room without one.'

'All right, all right.' I can tell Dr Shorland is annoyed. 'I'll give you a note. You realise how serious this is?'

'Yes, I do. I knew something was badly wrong when I saw her at school. But Mr Morrison told me it was all fine.'

Ah – *that* was where Mummy went when she came to see me in the sickbay. She went to see the headmaster. How brave she is.

'She told me you yourself tested her last term, Dr Shorland, and gave her a clean bill of health. And *he* told me…' It is as if Mummy is cutting each word out of ice and throwing it at the doctor. 'He told me that Lucy was making it all up, that she was trying to get people's sympathy because…because her own family doesn't love her.' I hear a stifled sob. 'You have a great deal to answer for.'

Two hours later, I'm lying on the back seat of a car with my head in Mummy's lap. I can smell Daddy's cigarette – it's funny how nice it smells, when Mrs Joyce's smelled so horrid – and overhead there floats a low murmur of voices. I feel warm and safe for the first time in ages. Slowly, I drift off to sleep.

*

'Where am I?'

'Shh, it's all right, darling. Daddy's got you.' I feel the familiar scratchy texture of his coat sleeve under my cheek.

'Where are we?'

'At the hospital. We're going to see Mr Atkins, the eye doctor – you like him, don't you?' That's Mummy's voice. I'm safe.

A nurse puts me to bed and gives me a drink of warm milk from a funny cup with a spout like a teapot. 'Good girl, that's right,' she says. 'Your mummy and daddy will be back to see you before you go to sleep.'

In a moment, they come in, and Mummy holds my hands tight. 'I'll be back to see you tomorrow afternoon after you've had your little operation, and Daddy will come and see you on Sunday. Be a good girl for Mummy, and try to lie very, very still.' She bends down and kisses me.

'Night-night, little one,' says Daddy. He kisses me too, and then they are gone.

I am in a side ward, and Mummy is sitting on the bed, holding both of my hands in hers.

'They told me that when they tried to put the mask on your face for the anaesthetic, you screamed at them not to hit you. Why was that, darling?'

Whenever I told them there was something wrong, they hit me.

'Come on, Lucy, darling, please tell Mummy what's upsetting you. Please, please, Lucy.'

At last, I feel large tears begin to roll down my face. I am sobbing and shaking. 'I won't have to go back there, Mummy, will I?' I whisper.

'No, darling – whatever happens, you'll never, never have to go back there again.'

Now the words tumble over each other as I try to describe the nightmare of the past few months: having to go to the toilet in the dark, the fall down the stairs, the beatings, the fall out of the van. 'Mrs Parker shouted at me and hit me. And so did Mrs Pryce. But it was true what I said, Mummy. I didn't tell lies, I didn't. I didn't!' Eventually, exhausted, I lie still and the darkness gathers around me. 'I love you, Mummy.'

'I love you too, darling. I love you too.'

I feel tears splash onto the backs of my hands.

Later on, I learn that I suffered a detached retina in my seeing eye as a result of the fall from the van. By the time I am seen by the eye surgeon, it is too late to do anything about it.

I am nine years old, and totally blind.

Part Two

1

I stay in the hospital in Cardiff for five weeks. A few days before I'm due to go home, the hospital almoner takes me out of the ward and into a nearby park. She buys us both an ice-cream cornet and we sit on the grass. The smell reminds me of our garden at home. I turn my cornet slowly, slowly, licking the soft, sweet ice cream.

'Would you like to make a daisy chain?' asks the almoner.

I crunch up the last little bit of my cornet. 'How?'

'Here, let me show you.' I hear the almoner shifting around on the grass, and then she tips the handful of daisies that she's picked into my lap. 'You hold one of the flowers like this,' she says, placing a stalk between my finger and thumb. 'Then you make a slit in the stem with your thumbnail. Now pick up another daisy from your lap, and thread it through the slit. That's right, clever girl. Then you make another slit in the second daisy and pick up the next one.'

Ten minutes later I've made a chain long enough to go around my neck.

The morning that I'm going home, one of the nurses washes my hair for me in the bath, then helps me get dressed in my new going-home clothes. 'Here's a pretty blue jumper,' she says, 'and a lovely cherry-red pinafore dress. And look – Sister's found a velvet ribbon for your hair. It's the same colour as your new dress. You'll look so smart for them all at home.'

I can feel the softness of the jumper as I slide my arms into the sleeves. I run my fingertips over the fine cord lines of the pinafore dress.

Sister Phillips brushes my hair gently but thoroughly, then winds the ringlets around her finger. 'There,' she says as she ties a bow in the ribbon. 'What a smart-looking girl you are.' I hear her give a little sigh as she turns away.

I feel excited. But I also feel scared.

'Baby,' I whisper in her ear – I'm hugging her with my right arm, and hanging on to the edge of the car seat with my left hand. 'It's strange in the car now that I can't see.'

I sway as the car turns a corner. I can hear other cars racing by, and a hissing, swishing sound that I realise after a while must be rain. I shiver and pull Baby even closer. Then comes the feeling I've been dreading: a churning in my stomach; a faintness. I must not be sick. I can't be sick in this kind woman's car. But a wave of bile races up my throat, and there is nothing whatever I can do to stop it.

2

When I wake up the next day I'm completely confused. The bed I'm in doesn't feel like my bed, and I can't hear the nurses. Then I hear the front door slam. That must be Stephen and Rosemary going off to school. I'm home, I'm home.

Mummy comes into the bedroom. 'Wakey-wakey, lazybones,' she calls out, and keeps up an incessant chatter while she helps me get dressed. 'What shall we do today?' she asks, and then, without waiting for an answer, 'How about going to the park?'

'Can't we stay at home?'

'Of course, darling, if that's what you'd like.' I hear her opening and shutting drawers; moving things around. Suddenly she asks, 'Have you been to the bathroom?'

No, I haven't. I'm too scared to go out onto the landing. I might go the wrong way and crash down the stairs.

'Never mind, we'll go now, before breakfast.'

For breakfast we have cornflakes.

'You can wear Mummy's apron,' says Mummy.

She ties it around my neck. I'm not a baby. But then, I might spill the milk and mess up my clothes...

Non-stop chatter, even while she's doing the washing-up. As if silence would be unbearable. 'Mummy'll have to go and fetch the dirty washing now. You can sit in Daddy's armchair and listen to the wireless while I do the washing.'

I listen to the familiar sounds of washday with *Housewives' Choice* in the background. First the *glug-glug* of water as the copper is filled. Then the *swish-swish* as the sheets are stirred with the copper stick.

'I could do with a cuppa,' says Mummy, 'while we wait for the copper to boil. Would you like a glass of milk and a Welsh cake?'

By dinner time, the house is filled with washday's steamy, soapy smells. I begin to feel something unclench inside me. Mummy is being a bit strange, but I'm home at last. I'm safe.

Soon a routine is established. I learn how to get dressed without help: how to feel for the front and the back of my vests and knickers; the bow at the front of a petticoat; the label at the back of a jumper. But somehow the front pockets of my pinafore dress too often end up over my bottom. On Tuesday and Thursday mornings we cross the humped bridge and walk to the farmhouse where Mummy has a cleaning job. For three hours I sit in the kitchen with the wireless on. Sometimes I want to scream with the boredom. On Wednesday afternoons we walk to Mr Jennings's corner store to do the shopping. At least there are interesting smells: cheese, bacon, tea, onions, and earthy potatoes, just like Daddy's. Mr Jennings often gives me a Toffee Cup. Other women chat to Mummy about the weather, or how their children are doing at school. No one ever asks when I'm going back to school.

I feel sort of happy, and settled, I suppose, but then one day, when Mummy is upstairs making the beds, I suddenly get this urge to move; to walk on my own without somebody leading me. I decide to try to walk around the living room. I stand up and put Baby in Daddy's armchair. Then I put out my left hand and slide it along the brass rail at the top of the fireguard. I creep forwards.

My knees bump against the soft edge of Mummy's armchair. I turn and slide my hand along the wall until I hit the back of a chair pushed in under the table – my chair. Then Stephen's, then Rosemary's, and then I turn left to face Mummy's chair. I lean over and reach out to touch the back of Daddy's chair, pressed up against the wall. Turning again, I touch the windowsill and the wooden arm of the bed settee. I shuffle sideways along the front of it. Next comes a short section of wall; then nothing. Empty space. For a moment I can't think; I'm so terrified my mind goes blank, then I realise: it's the kitchen doorway. I take a deep breath, count to three, and plunge across the gap, bumping my head on the doorpost on the other side. Ow!

Then I mutter, 'Sideboard,' and feel for the two brass candlesticks. I jump as the second one clatters onto its side. I stand it up again.

Now I've reached Daddy's desk; I run my fingers over the raised pattern on the sloped panel to find the keyhole. Then I am back at his armchair.

'I did it, Baby.' I snatch her up and give her a cuddle. 'I did it all by myself.'

3

We're in the grocer's one Wednesday afternoon when a woman comes in whom Mummy hasn't met before. Mr Jennings introduces her as Mrs Gordon. She is a widow with two girls who have grown up and left home, and she now lives alone. She tells Mummy that she often feels lonely, and then asks her if she could possibly lend me to her once a week, perhaps on one of the mornings when Mummy's out at her cleaning job?

Mummy doesn't reply at once. 'But…' she says after a moment, and then hurriedly, almost under her breath, 'Lucy is blind.'

It is obvious to me that Mrs Gordon knew this already.

So begins the enchantment of Thursday mornings. They always follow the same pattern. After breakfast, we take Stephen and Rosemary to catch the school bus, and then after just a few more steps we arrive at Mrs Gordon's house. The door always opens just as Mummy rings the bell.

The first morning, Mrs Gordon says, 'Hello, Lucy, you're just in time to help me wind up all the clocks. We'll do the bedroom clock first.'

Hand in hand, we climb the thickly carpeted stairs, counting the steps aloud. 'One, two, three…fourteen – turn left on the small landing. Fifteen…twenty.'

A few more paces and we're in the big bedroom, and Mrs Gordon shows me a little clock that stands on a glass-topped dressing table with silky curtains. It makes a funny whirring noise as she winds it up.

Every week it is the same routine. The tinkly bell of the bedroom clock always begins to chime nine as we start down the stairs. The grandmother clock stands at the turn. This too begins to chime the hour. Its silvery tones follow us down to the hall, where the tall grandfather clock bongs in deeper tones. My favourite is the clock that stands on the sideboard in the dining room. Its shiny wooden case is nice to stroke, and a cool metal band runs around the glass. Mrs Gordon opens the glass for me, and, taking care not to move the hands, I run the tips of my fingers over the raised numbers. This clock plays two tunes. One is like Big Ben on the wireless, but it's the other I like best. Mrs Gordon tells me it's called the 'Whittington Chimes': *Turn again, Whittington, Lord Mayor of London*.

The last clock is a small brass carriage clock on the sitting-room mantelpiece. It sits next to a framed photo, which Mrs Gordon tells me is of her husband with their two girls when they were small. He is wearing military uniform. A red paper poppy sits in front of the photograph.

Here is where the piano lives. I've seen a piano before, but I've never touched one. We sit down in front of it. Mrs Gordon lifts the lid and plays a few notes, and then she picks up my hands and places my fingers on the keys. Now that her girls have left home, no one plays this piano. In the weeks to come Mrs Gordon will show me how to play some simple tunes, and with her encouragement I begin to pick out one or two of the hymns that we sing in church. I always practise while Mrs Gordon is out in the kitchen preparing a tray with drinks and biscuits: coffee for her; orange squash for me.

And then, my favourite part of the morning: we settle down, with me on a fat round pouffe leaning against the arm of Mrs Gordon's chair, and she reads to me. That first Thursday, she chooses to begin *The Wind in the Willows* with me. She tells me that her two girls used to love it when they were about my age. For the whole of the next week I am longing to get back to the River Bank; to climb into a little boat and gently scull past the rushes and the reeds with my new friends Ratty and Mole.

4

The months pass. Every so often, out of the corner of my ear, I overhear Mummy and Daddy, when they think I'm not listening, use words like 'negligence', 'suing' and 'lawyers', as well as some other words and phrases – 'irreversible' and 'totally avoidable' – that are attached to the word 'blindness'. These conversations make me want to cry, but I can't cry or they'll know I've been listening to them talking.

And now a social worker called Miss Briggs enters our lives. She is trying to find me a new school, according to Mummy. But I don't want to go to a new school. I don't want to go to any school ever again. But I am beginning to feel bored at home.

One afternoon, I go to the toy cupboard to get out my old books and comics. I put my hands right to the back of the cupboard, but I can't feel them anywhere.

'They're no good to you any more,' says Mummy when I ask her where they are. 'I thought some other little girl would like to have them.'

'But they're mine,' I cry. 'They're mine! They're mine!'

Mummy tries to hug me. 'But, darling, you can't read them any more.'

I wriggle out of her arms and plunge back into the toy cupboard, and come out clutching a paintbox and a large painting book. Defiantly, I tell her, 'I'm going to paint a picture.'

I stumble past the table and the settee, open the kitchen door, then stumble through and out past the closed pantry. I reach the back door and pull it open. I step out, turn right, and follow the painted brick passage to the side door. I run the back of my hand along the brickwork, turn right again, stop by the open front door, and sink down on the threshold. I've never made that journey since coming back from hospital, but I realise now that it is all clear in my head. I can see every step of the way.

And here's Mummy on the doorstep with a wooden kitchen chair, which she sets down in front of me, with a jam jar full of water.

All afternoon I sit and splodge patches of colour onto the paper. A parade of colours passes inside my head: red and yellow; pink and green; purple, orange and blue. I'll see them again one day.

When Stephen gets home from school he offers me some Smarties. 'Because you've been sad, Lucy,' he says. He asks what colour I'd like, and I tell him green and red. A rattle as he shakes the box; then he picks up my hand and places five Smarties on my palm. 'Three green and two red,' he tells me.

Later, I overhear Mummy and Daddy in the kitchen. Daddy sounds cross.

'I told you not to give them away, Mary.'

'But, Jack, they're no use to her now.'

'I know, I know, darling, but you still shouldn't have given them away. They belonged to Lucy. They weren't yours to give.'

5

'It's your turn now, Lucy,' says Stephen. 'You need a five or a three.'

I finger the dots on my dominoes, and shake my head. 'No good.'

'Then you must give a knock,' says Stephen.

I tap a domino on the table.

The kitchen door opens. It's Dan. He's engaged to be married to Cousin Jill, who's now training to be a nurse. 'I'm not stopping,' he says. 'I'm going for a drink with Jill, but I've brought something for Lucy.'

'What is it?' I ask, putting down the domino I'm holding.

'It's a pack of cards,' says Stephen.

'Sort of,' Dan says. 'But they've got letters on them. Hold out your hand, Lucy.' He places a card in my hand. 'So, what letter's that?'

'There's sandpaper on it,' Stephen says excitedly. 'It looks like the—'

Dan shushes him. They are both quiet as I feel the card.

'It's a big sandpaper "A".'

'Clever girl,' says Dan. 'Now, if you move your finger around a bit, you'll find something else.'

'It's round, like a rough dot from one of my dominoes.'

'That's right, Lucy: it's a letter "A" in Braille. Braille is how people who can't see read books. Here's a box with nine more letters and their Braille dots. See if you can tell Stephen what the letters are. Then perhaps you can begin to learn the Braille letters too. Must run now, or Jill will think I'm not coming.'

We abandon the dominoes and play with the cards for the rest of the evening.

'This one's a big "D". It's a stick joined to a backwards "C".'

'And this one?' Stephen hands me another card.

I run my fingers over the sandpaper. 'It's a big "H".'

'Let's make words with them,' suggests Stephen. 'How about "bed"?'

I sift through the cards, looking for the right letters until I find 'B', 'E' and 'D'.

'I wonder if I could do that with my eyes closed?' says Stephen. And then, 'Oh, it feels funny.'

'The dots don't look like the letters we know,' I say. 'There's one for "A" and two for "B", but there's two for "C" too.'

'And for "E" and "I",' says Stephen.

I feel the cards again. 'But they're different. "A" is one dot, "B" is two straight down, and for "C" they're side by side.'

That night I take the cards up to bed with me. I feel as if a little door has opened in my mind, but I don't know what's on the other side of it. Sandpaper letters dance through my dreams.

6

Miss Briggs comes round one day to tell us that she has found what she thinks would be a suitable school for me: a small boarding school for blind children with other handicaps. It's called Brilbeck House, and it's in Herefordshire. Mummy and Daddy insist that they see the school before they agree to send me there.

Thinking about it later, I will realise that this must have taken some courage on their part. Deference to authority was hardwired into people in those days in class-bound England, but they had learned wariness from what had happened to me at Hinton Grange, and determination that nothing like that would happen again.

Daddy's been given the day off so that he can come with us. Miss Briggs is driving, with Daddy beside her in the passenger seat.

'A fine day for a drive in the country,' Miss Briggs burbles as we set off.

Sitting on the back seat next to Mummy, I stay quiet. Myself, I'd rather stay at home.

We're not due at the school until the afternoon, so we stop off for lunch at a roadside café. The fish and chips are nice, but it's horrid chasing peas around.

'There are more peas at the back of your plate,' says Daddy helpfully.

I try to scoop them up with my spoon.

'They're at nine o'clock now,' he says. 'Oh, well done – you've got two, but five of them have escaped to seven o'clock.'

I try again, but when the spoon reaches my mouth it is empty. I feel my eyes fill with tears.

'Never mind, darling – let Mummy get them for you. Open sesame!'

I open my mouth and she spoons the peas in.

'There, all gone.'

My face has gone hot. Miss Briggs suggests cake for pudding, and I'm grateful to her.

It's not much further to the school, but the road turns into a rutted country lane, which soon starts to climb, and my tummy begins to churn. The car swings to the right, then to the left, and comes to a stop just as I puke up all my lunch.

'It's all right, darling,' says Mummy. She takes a damp flannel from the shopping bag at her feet, and wipes my face. 'There's a clean cardie in my bag, so it doesn't matter.'

We get out and Daddy takes my hand and counts out loud as we climb two short flights of wide, shallow steps. The front door is open, and we go in. Our shoes make a loud noise on the wooden floor.

Someone comes out from a room off to the right, and introduces himself as Mr Stewart, the headmaster. 'Are you all right, Lucy? You're looking rather pale.'

'She's just been sick in the car,' says Miss Briggs.

'Oh dear – would you like to lie down and have a little sleep, Lucy?'

I hang on tight to Daddy's hand. No way. If I do that, when I wake up they'll have gone home without me.

'Never mind,' says Mr Stewart. 'Silly me. Let's go to my office for a cup of tea and a chat instead.'

I think he sounds nice. He tells us that there are seventy children at Brilbeck House, all of them with various kinds of sight problems and other handicaps. Then he suggests that we visit the library, where some children are being read to by a teacher, who is introduced as Miss Browning. She suggests I stay and listen to the story while the headmaster continues to show Mummy and Daddy around.

'You'd like to hear a story, wouldn't you, Lucy?' Miss Browning asks.

'Yes, but Mummy and Daddy will come back soon, won't they?'

'Of course, darling. We won't be long,' says Daddy, and he ruffles my hair.

Don't they know how scared I am? I wonder.

'Come and sit next to me,' says the teacher, 'then you'll hear better. We're reading *Rikki-Tikki-Tavi*.'

I've never heard of it, but it's a really good story; kind of exciting. Mummy and Daddy reappear soon after the story is finished and the other children have gone off somewhere else. Miss Browning wants to know if I am learning Braille.

'No, not exactly,' Mummy tells her, 'but a friend has made her some cards with letters and dots on.'

She shows them to Miss Browning, who, after a moment or two, says, 'The dots are much too big – that's no good.'

But they're mine. My very own lovely, proper letters. Daddy squeezes my hand.

I feel exhausted. As I drift off to sleep in the car on the way home, my dreams mingle with the low murmur of voices above me.

'The headmaster seems kind… *Rikki-Tikki-Tavi*… Nag the snake…blind teacher… Miss Browning…unusual… Darzee the tailorbird…'

7

I'm told that we have to wait to hear whether Mr Stewart is going to offer me a place at Brilbeck House. I hope he won't. I don't want to leave home, with its weekly routine that I love. As if it's a magic spell, I sometimes chant quietly to myself, 'Monday: washday, Tuesday: farmhouse, Wednesday: corner shop…' Thursdays are best: down by the River Bank with Mrs Gordon, Ratty, Mole and Toad. 'Friday: clean the house.'

Then one Monday, after dinner, Mummy announces, 'Miss Briggs is bringing someone to see you later this afternoon.'

'To see *me*? Why?'

'She's a teacher. As you're not at school just now, she's coming here to give you lessons.'

'What's she like?'

'I don't know. I haven't met her yet, but I'm sure she'll be nice. Her name's Miss Armstrong. She can't see, like you, and she has a dog.'

A dog. That sounds nice. But even so, what if this new teacher shouts like Mrs Parker, or – horrible thought – hits me?

At four o'clock, Miss Armstrong arrives with Sheba, her dog. Mummy tells me to sit next to Miss Armstrong on the sofa while she brings through the tea tray.

Miss Armstrong says, 'I hope, Lucy, that you and I are going to be friends?'

I don't know what to say to that, so I say nothing.

'I used to teach another little girl, called Jackie.'

'My daddy's called Jack.'

'And what is your mummy's name?'

'Mary.'

'That's a nice name. My name is Edith. Now, show me your hands, Lucy.'

I hold them out and feel them being held and gently stroked.

Miss Armstrong says nothing about my bent fingers or my knobbly knuckles. Instead she asks me if I like reading stories, so I tell her, 'I can't read any more.' And then I add, speaking very quietly because I'm not sure if the door to the kitchen is open or shut, that Mummy's given all my books away. 'Even *Heidi*, which was my best story.'

'Well,' says Miss Armstrong, 'that's why I'm here. I can't see, just like you, but I read lots and lots of books.'

'Books with dots?'

'Yes – how do you know about our dots?'

'Jill's friend Dan made me some cards with proper letters and dots on them.'

'I see. Will you show them to me?'

'You won't take them away, will you?'

'No, I promise not to take them away.'

'I've hidden them here.' I stand up and lift the cushion beneath me, and hand over to Miss Armstrong my box of letter cards.

'This is very clever of Dan, but our dots are much smaller,' says Miss Armstrong, and she hands back the box.

I put it back under the cushion, just in case.

'I've got a book with me. Would you like to try some of our dots?'

'Mmm.'

She tells me she is putting a book on the table, and then she takes one of my hands and places my index finger at the beginning of a line. 'Try moving your finger along to the right.'

'Lots of tiny dots. Will I ever be able to read them?'

'Of course, once you've learned how. And now, shall I read you a story?'

'Yes, please.'

I feel a soft, warm head under my hand, and as I squeeze myself a bit closer to Miss Armstrong on the sofa, Sheba settles herself against my legs and lays her head in my lap. Gently, I stroke her silky ears.

Now every day – washday, shop day, River Bank day, cleaning day – leads towards four o'clock and the arrival of Miss Armstrong and Sheba. First I learn how to use a Braillette board, with its holes and pegs for making Braille dots. I learn that the holes are in groups of six, called cells, with one letter for each cell. In the first lesson we do the first ten letters, and Miss Armstrong writes some words for me to read out.

'"Heidi".' That makes me smile. '"Bead bag". "Deaf egg".' I giggle. 'Eggs don't have ears to hear anyway.'

'That was very good. Now I'll write the next ten letters for you. See how many you can learn before I come tomorrow.'

Ten letters a day. But Miss Armstrong's books don't have any pictures. I want my old books back, I tell her, and I burst into tears.

'I'm sorry, Lucy, but I can't give you them back. Come on now, you're doing really well, and soon you'll be able to have lots of books with new stories. That will be good, won't it?'

'I just want things to be like they used to be. I don't like it in the dark.'

'That's the way it is, and we have to make the best of it. Now dry your eyes and get on with learning,' says Miss Armstrong.

Each afternoon, Monday to Friday, Miss Armstrong arrives at four and lessons begin. After the alphabet, I have to learn the contractions, and then the letters that are used for whole words. Then she says it's time for me to start writing Braille, which, she explains, has to be done backwards. At first I don't understand.

She gives me the Braillette board. 'Write "I am Lucy Holland" on it.'

I put the pegs in the holes, and Miss Armstrong checks them.

'Very good, Lucy. You've got it absolutely perfect. Let's close the lid and click it shut. Now, I'm going to turn it over, and you can feel the other end of the pegs. Remember they're rather sharp.'

I run my fingers over the ends of the pegs, puzzled. 'It doesn't make sense.'

'No,' agrees Miss Armstrong, 'because it's upside down and backwards. We need to be able to do this on paper. Then when we turn it over, it will read all right again.'

'How can we do that?'

'We use a hand frame and a stylus,' replies Miss Armstrong. 'Here, I'll show you. The frame has a board, a clamp to hold the paper, two rows of cells, and a stylus. Let's put a sheet of paper in the clamp.' She gives me a short needle with a wooden handle. 'Press the point down on the paper through the holes in the cells, and you will feel a little crunch as you make a dot. Play with the frame over the weekend. Then when I come on Monday, we'll see what you've done. Try writing from right to left instead of left to right. You can move the cells down when you want to do two more rows.'

Sheba pushes her cold nose into my hand to say goodbye. I think she's also wishing me good luck.

At night in bed, I repeat to myself, '"B" is "but", "C" is "can", "D" is "do", "ABV" is "above", "WD" is "would"…' Visions of the real letters float before my eyes, lulling me to sleep.

Days and weeks pass. July comes, and Stephen and Rosemary are at home all day. It's only me who still has lessons. The Taylor frame joins the hand frame on the small parlour table, and I learn Braille arithmetic: the rows of small octagonal holes can be turned into numbers by the special use of pegs.

'Look, Lucy,' Miss Armstrong says. 'At one end of the pegs there's a bar which becomes "one" to "eight", depending on the angle you put them in the holes. The two points at the other end become "nine" and "zero", or "plus", "minus", "divide", "multiply" or "equals" – isn't that clever?'

Lying in bed one night, swapping between the litany of letters and the dance of numbers, I suddenly realise how much I love my lessons with Miss Armstrong, and how, every night when I go to bed, I'm already looking forward to what I'm going to learn the next day.

8

At the beginning of August, Mummy tells me that I have to go with her and Daddy to a meeting with a new firm of solicitors in Coventry, about our claim for negligence against Hinton Grange and the county council. Later I'll discover – Mummy doesn't explain it to me now, and perhaps she doesn't fully understand it herself – why we have to go all the way to Coventry. The original solicitors, it transpires, who are based close by in Warwick, also do work for the county council. There is a conflict of interest. Why was this not made clear earlier? I realise later that precious time was lost.

'The gentleman we're going to see will want to talk to you about what happened at Hinton Grange,' Mummy tells me.

'I don't want to talk about that.'

'I know, darling,' says Daddy, 'but we need to try and help other little girls to not have accidents.'

It takes three separate buses to get to Coventry. All the way there, I feel sick with dread.

The lawyer is called Mr Dean. He starts by asking Mummy to describe what happened. She tells him about coming to see me at Hinton Grange at the end of February, and finding me in the sickbay; about how I didn't recognise her when she came in; about how I couldn't see the difference in colour between the wrappers on my favourite chocolate bars. Then she tells him about how she went to find the headmaster, to ask him how long I hadn't been able to see, and Mr Morrison told her that I wasn't really blind, and that I was just pretending so as to cover up other things, such as…that Mummy didn't love me.

Mummy starts crying, and that makes me cry too, and I reach out for her hand and say, 'Don't cry, Mummy, please don't cry.'

I don't want to talk about it at all, but Mr Dean says it's important, that I must, and because he sounds nice I find myself telling him about the falls I had, about being scared of the dark corridor but even more scared of what would happen if I wet the bed, about the stile and the barbed wire, about falling over the milk crate, and about having to stand up in the van, and falling out of it when the door wasn't closed properly.

In the middle of August, Miss Armstrong goes away for a week's holiday, and leaves me with my first real Braille book to read. It's only a *Dick and Dora* story and it's not very interesting, but I can read it all by myself, and I do so over and over. I'm really looking forward to when Miss Armstrong comes back so that I can ask her for other books.

But then one evening, unannounced, Miss Briggs turns up. My heart sinks when I hear her voice. I'm sent out into the garden with Stephen and Rosemary while she talks to Mummy and Daddy, and when I'm called back in on my own I know that what I fear most has happened. I have been offered a place at Brilbeck House, to start halfway through September. Miss Briggs has persuaded Mummy and Daddy that this is a wonderful opportunity for me, and that we can 'put the past behind us' and 'look to the future'.

That night, I cry myself to sleep.

9

'We'll do the clocks first, as usual,' says Mrs Gordon.

All the clocks are saying, *Goodbye, goodbye, goodbye.*

'You're very quiet today, Lucy,' Mrs Gordon says.

Suddenly, tears are coursing down my cheeks. 'I'm going away,' I sob.

'Going away? Where to?'

'School. It's called Brilbeck House.'

'I see.' She takes my hand in hers. 'But you'll be back for Christmas.'

'That's a long way away. You'll have forgotten me by then.'

She kneels and puts an arm around me. 'No, no, Lucy – I'll never, ever forget you.' She gets up. 'Wait a minute, I'll be back.' She returns a few minutes later. 'Here,' she says, and places a large doll on my lap. 'I was wondering if you could look after Gwenny for me? You see, she's very lonely now that my girls have gone away. I'm sure she would like to have another little girl to look after her. Do you think you could do that for me?'

'I expect so,' I murmur.

'That's good, but Gwenny will get upset if she sees you crying.'

I pull my hanky out of my sleeve and dry my eyes. 'I'll try to be good.'

'Do you think Gwenny would like to meet our friends down by the River Bank?'

I nod, and try to smile.

Soon the clocks begin to chime half past twelve, and it's time to go home.

'I'll get your coat,' Mrs Gordon says, 'and Gwenny's shawl.'

Every night now I cry myself to sleep, hugging Gwenny close and murmuring, 'Sorry, Gwenny, I'll try to be good, I will,' but somehow the tears keep coming.

Sometimes I hear snatches of conversation from downstairs.

'I don't like Lucy going away again so soon.' Daddy's voice. 'She's settled and happy at the moment, and she's doing all right with Miss Armstrong, isn't she?'

'If we turn down this place we might have to wait two years or more to get Lucy back into school.' Mummy's voice.

Daddy: 'We thought she'd be safe at the other school, and look what happened.'

The days fly by, as though racing to be rid of me. I hate saying goodbye. So many people to say goodbye to before I go: the people at Sunday school; Miss Armstrong; Mr Jennings at the shop; Jill and Dan, who are soon going to get married; Rosemary and Stephen; Aunt Renée and Uncle Bill; and, worst of all, Daddy. I'm taking Gwenny with me, but I tell Rosemary that Baby has said she wants to stay at home, so I ask Rosemary to look after her.

Rosemary grabs her and jumps up and down, shouting, 'Baby, Baby, my Baby.'

The day comes, and once again I'm sitting next to Mummy in the back of Miss Briggs's car, driving away from home to Brilbeck House. I feel strange inside, as though I'm not really here, and my tummy's full of groans and grumbles. It's a nightmare journey. I am sick three times.

'Here at last,' says Miss Briggs, making a sharp turn.

In the wood-floored hall, we are greeted by a woman who introduces herself as Miss Honeybourne. 'Hello, Lucy.' She has a kind, motherly voice. 'I'm going to be your new family mother here at school. Tea's over, but we've saved some especially for you.'

I shake my head.

'She was very sick in the car,' says Mummy.

'Oh dear – well, perhaps just some warm milk, then?' Miss Honeybourne leads the way upstairs, and opens a door into a dormitory. 'This is your bed, Lucy,' she says. 'The third along on the right.'

Soon I am tucked in, with Gwenny beside me.

'Be a good girl for Mummy.' Mummy bends over and kisses me on the forehead. 'Daddy and I will be back to see you very soon. Goodbye, darling. Be good for Mummy now.'

I hear her footsteps retreat and the dormitory door click shut. I lie rigid with Gwenny folded tightly in my arms, too exhausted even to cry much. Just a few tears ooze from under my eyelids. Then I plunge down a dark tunnel into unconsciousness and sleep.

10

Slowly, I drift up into consciousness. Someone is holding my hand and stroking it gently.

'Wakey-wakey, lazybones,' says a soft voice. 'It's time to get up, Lucy.'

I snap awake. I'm not at home. I'm at school. My eyes fill and overflow.

'Oh dear,' Miss Honeybourne says. 'Let's put your dressing gown and slippers on and go to the bathroom. You'll feel better when you're washed and dressed. Then we'll go to breakfast – you must be hungry.'

Back in the dormitory, I get dressed.

'Now I'll do your hair,' Miss Honeybourne says. 'Such pretty hair.' She brushes it gently, winding the ringlets around her fingers. 'There – you look very nice.' Then she takes my hand. 'We'll go this way, to the lift.'

'I want to take Gwenny,' I say, and fumble on the bed for her.

I think Miss Honeybourne is going to say no, but instead she says, 'Of course,' and puts Gwenny in my arms. Then, with a guiding hand on my shoulder, she leads the way out of the dormitory and along a gallery to the lift, and presses the button. *Ping.* The metal gates clank open. We step in, the gates shut, and the cage descends.

Soon I am surrounded by chattering children and clashing cutlery. I don't like it. I want to go home.

'Shall we sit Gwenny on the chair at the head of the table? Then she can watch us eat.'

Reluctantly, I let Miss Honeybourne take the doll from my arms.

'You must be hungry,' Miss Honeybourne says again as she sits down next to me. 'Do you like porridge?'

I nod. The smell of porridge and toast is making my mouth water. Suddenly, I do feel quite hungry.

It's nice porridge – not quite like Mummy's, but nice. And there's a nice crunchy sound as I eat the toast and scrambled eggs.

When breakfast is over, Miss Honeybourne takes me into the hall and sits me on a window seat. 'Ah, here's Mr Tapley, one of the teachers,' she says.

'You must be the new girl. Lucy, isn't it? Can I take your picture for the school album?'

I hold Gwenny tight, and nod my head.

'That's a nice dolly. What's her name?'

'Gwenny,' I whisper.

'Shall we have Gwenny in the picture too?'

Again, I nod, and then blink as the camera flashes. It's mostly dark for me now, but sometimes there are tiny reminders of seeing. I don't know whether to be glad about that, or extra sad.

'And here's Mr Swift,' says Miss Honeybourne. 'I'll leave you with him. See you at dinner time, Lucy.' Her footsteps retreat, and I am left with yet another stranger.

'Shall I show you round, Lucy?' asks Mr Swift. 'Can I carry your dolly for you?'

'No…no, thank you.' I tighten my grip on Gwenny.

We move down the hall and Mr Swift opens a door. 'This is the gym. We play all sorts of games in here.'

On the far side of the room, he places my hand on what feels like a fence. It's a bit like Daddy's chicken run, but stiffer. Then Mr Swift says something about canes, and my heart gives a lurch. Canes? This place is going to be as bad as Hinton Grange. I can't help it. I burst into tears.

'Lucy, what's wrong?' Mr Swift is kneeling beside me.

'Canes,' I sob. 'For hitting.'

'No, no, no, Lucy – I said *games*. This is the cage where we keep the balls for playing *games* with. Look, I'll show you.' He opens a gate in the fence and brings out a ball with a bell in it. 'Now, dry your eyes, or Miss Wakefield, your teacher, will be cross with me.'

'Sorry,' I whisper. 'Sorry, sorry.'

'That's all right,' he says, patting my shoulder. And then he adds, 'Nobody ever gets hit here.'

Later, I have my first Braille lesson with Miss Browning. She uses a Stainsby, which she tells me is easier to work with than the hand frame I've been using with Miss Armstrong. It has a board and a clamp just like a hand frame, but six round keys for the dots and a long bar to make spaces with. The carriage with the keys is moved to the right-hand end of the row. On each hand, the little finger and its neighbour make the top dots, the middle finger makes dots two and five, and the index finger makes dots three and six.

Miss Browning places my fingers on the keys and pushes them all down. 'Now, do me a row of all six dots.'

'A row of "for"s?'

'That's right, clever girl.'

I whisper, 'For, for, for,' each time I push the six keys down.

By teatime I am completely exhausted. I think I fall asleep at the table, because the next thing I know I'm being carried upstairs by Miss Honeybourne. She helps me undress and tucks me into bed with a cup of hot milk beside me.

Soon the pattern of the days becomes a welcome, familiar tread. Here at Brilbeck House, everyone learns in a different way. Some children don't do any reading and writing at all. Lots of them play the piano. There are a lot of pianos in the school – five at least – and they are in constant use.

I long to start piano lessons. I'm worried that I'll forget the notes that Mrs Gordon taught me. Meanwhile, the singing teacher has said that I should join the school choir, so as well as singing in class, I do choir practice after tea on Mondays and on Saturday mornings. At the harvest festival we sing 'We Plough the Fields and Scatter', and a picture flashes across my inner eye: a church windowsill decorated with a sheaf of corn in shades of green and yellow.

The memories of Hinton Grange are fading like ice melting in the sunshine. But there are things about this new school that still frighten me. Everyone seems bigger than me, and definitely noisier. When everyone else clatters into the hall, I turn in towards the wall, and tuck my toes into the corner so that no one steps on them. The other children's voices are loud, and yet at the same time oddly blurred. Often I can't quite catch what people are saying to me. They shout a lot, and I don't really think that they're shouting at me, but I'm not one hundred per cent sure about that.

11

The school doctor wants to send me to a hearing specialist at the hospital. I tell him that I don't like hospitals, and that I'd rather not go. He assures me that I won't have to stay; that I'll just need to see Dr Jacob and let her do a small test.

'Will you do that for me?' he asks.

They'll make me anyway. 'All right,' I say politely. 'As long as I don't have to stay.'

The appointment comes two weeks after my eleventh birthday. At the hospital – the tiled floors and swing doors are all too familiar to me, as is the sick-making smell of dinner and disinfectant all mixed up – the consultant comments on how pale I am (Miss Honeybourne explains that I was sick in the minibus on the way over), and then looks down my ears. No one has ever looked into my ears before. I have to do a test that involves putting on earphones and squeezing a rubber bulb whenever I hear a noise. Some of the bleeps and beeps are loud and shrill, others rumble like foghorns, and some are so faint that I have to strain to catch them. It's quite fun squeezing the bulb, and I'm sorry when the test is over.

A few days later, Miss Honeybourne takes me to the headmaster's office because he has something to tell me. In that office I learn that I have no useful hearing in my right ear, and a degree of hearing loss in my left. I am going to have to use a hearing aid.

What I don't know until much later, when one day Mum inadvertently lets it slip, is that some of the staff at Brilbeck House were wondering then whether it would be better if I were moved into the Annexe, the small facility next door for deaf-blind children. Looking back, I think that it was probably thanks to Miss Honeybourne and my class teacher, Miss Wakefield, that I wasn't transferred. Thank you, Miss Honeybourne. Thank you, Miss Wakefield. My life would have been very different.

12

That Christmas, Mum and Dad (now I'm more grown-up this is what I call them) give me a recorder, and at the beginning of the spring term I join Mr Swift's Thursday evening recorder group.

More than ever, I long to have piano lessons. Everyone else in my class plays the piano, but when I ask Miss Wakefield, she says she thinks I wouldn't manage it with my bent fingers. 'And aren't you enjoying your recorder lessons?' she asks.

At the end of January I am fitted with a hearing aid for my left ear. I go to the hospital to have a mould made, and return three weeks later to be given the odd-shaped lump of plastic that from now on I'll have to wear inside my ear. It doesn't hurt, but as I hold the plastic lump in my hand and turn it over between my fingers, I can't see how it's going to help me hear.

'You're a smart girl and I expect you'll get used to it in no time,' says Dr Jacob briskly. 'I'm going to give your hearing aid to Miss Honeybourne, and when you're back at school Mr Stewart will show you how it works. As everything's settled, I'll not see you for a while…' She pauses. 'But before you go, how about a sherbet lemon? I think they're your favourite sweets, is that right?'

I nod.

'Open your mouth.' She pops a sweet onto my tongue, then presses the rest of the bag into my hand.

I mumble, 'Thank you,' thinking that Mum would be upset by my talking with my mouth full. It makes me giggle.

There's obviously more to this hearing aid than I realised. On the way back in the school minibus, Miss Honeybourne gives me the rest of the device to hold: a chunky square bag that sprouts wires.

The next day, instead of going to lessons when the two o'clock bell rings, I go to Mr Stewart's office.

'Now, Lucy,' he says, 'let's put it on.' And he slips the strap of the shoulder bag over my head, sliding it under my left arm. 'At the end of the thick wire there are two bits like press studs that join the lead to the batteries, and I've put them in the bag. Here's the speaker.' He clips it to the strap across my chest. 'Next we need to put in the ear mould.' He drapes the thin wire over my right shoulder and around my neck, and gently pushes the mould into my ear.

Sitting very still, I wonder what will happen next.

A faint click makes me jump, and Mr Stewart asks, 'Can you hear me, Lucy?'

I say, 'Yes,' and jump again at the loudness of my own voice.

'Here's the volume,' says Mr Stewart, and he places my finger on a knurled switch. It feels like the edge of a shilling or a sixpence. 'I'm going to talk, and I want you to move the knob until my voice sounds comfortable: not too loud, or too quiet. Is that all right?'

'Yes.' Wow, much too loud; I turn the knob hard.

'…lessons did you do this morning?'

'Ouch!' His voice hits my eardrum.

'Move it the other way.'

'Too quiet.'

'Try moving it just a tiny bit.'

'That's better.'

For the next week I spend fifteen minutes every day with Mr Stewart, practising: learning how to not talk so loudly that my own voice hurts my ear; how to move the ridged knob very, very gently; how to keep changing it whenever anything, such as Mr Stewart's telephone, is suddenly too loud.

On Friday, he says, 'Next week, we'll go around the school together and try the hearing aid in different places.'

First we visit Miss Honeybourne in the sewing room. She provides lemonade and ginger nuts, but a knock at the door hits my ear so hard that I spill my lemonade. Both of the grown-ups tell me not to worry, and Miss Honeybourne quickly refills my glass. Then we visit Miss Browning in the library, who asks me to read out a short passage from the book we've been reading in library hour, *Five Children and It*.

'Well done!' she says when I stop, and Mr Stewart repeats, 'Yes, well done!'

I wear the aid to assembly at the end of the week, and when the whole school sings 'Onward, Christian Soldiers', I almost have to turn it right off.

I wear the aid every day: for a few hours at first, and then for longer periods. I slowly get used to the way the bag slaps against my thigh as I walk. What's really difficult to deal with is the way the wires catch on door handles and the backs of chairs, pulling me up suddenly as I walk by. Every night I put the bag, wires and mould into the locker next to my bed, and soon I feel as though I'm not properly dressed until I've pushed the mould into my left ear in the morning and switched it on. By the Easter holidays the hearing aid has become just another part of my daily routine.

13

School holidays are very different now from when I was at Hinton Grange. It's lovely to be at home: to play in the garden with Stephen and Rosemary; to play dominoes with Dad in the evenings; to let Mum spoil me with my favourite meals, and with Welsh cakes or ginger nuts every teatime. But I don't dread going back to school. In fact, I look forward to it: perhaps soon they'll let me have piano lessons.

So it comes as a horrible shock when, one afternoon when Jill has taken Stephen and Rosemary out to the park, Mum tells me without preamble that after Easter I am going back to the Coventry hospital for what she calls 'another little operation' on my legs.

'No, no!' I cry out. 'Please, no! I don't want another operation.'

'I know, love, but if you're a good girl and have your little op, Daddy and I will give you a Braille watch.'

I slump onto the settee, not even trying to control my sobbing. They'll make me do it anyway. Grown-ups can always make you do what they want.

'We need you to do this,' says Mum.

'Will I be able to tell the time with the Braille watch?'

'Yes – it's just like the watch Miss Armstrong showed you one day, don't you remember?' Then, as if she wants to get all the bad things out of the way in one go, Mum goes on, 'Lucy, I need to read something to you.'

'What?'

'What you told the solicitor, Mr Dean. You remember, about what happened at Hinton Grange?'

'No!' I shout. 'No, no!'

'But we have to, so that you don't forget.'

'But I want to forget.'

'I know, darling, but we need to do this to help other children in the future. Now come on, Lucy. It won't take long and I'll make your favourite tea when we've finished.'

I try not to listen, but I can't shut out Mum's voice.

She begins, '"It was a Thursday…"'

I feel sick. It is as if it is happening all over again: the dark corridor and the stone stairs; Mrs Pryce shaking me; the horrible, crowded van, and having to stand squeezed in beside the door; Mrs Parker hitting me on my swollen knuckles… I want to shut it all out and never think of it again.

14

Coventry again, and once more I'm walking up the slope to the hospital entrance. I am eleven years old, and I can no longer see the entrance in front of me.

As before, I come round from the operation to find my legs encased in heavy plaster. But this time there is a watch – the promised Braille watch – waiting for me. I must be careful not to move the hands, I think as I pick it up and feel it.

I wake repeatedly throughout that night, and every time I wake, I reach over to my locker to feel for the small box that contains my very own watch.

This time round, I don't get to have lessons with the others on the ward. The teacher has said that she doesn't know 'how to teach the blind'. It is dull during the mornings with nobody to talk to and nothing to do. But Mum comes every afternoon and (telling me that this is in fact Mrs Gordon's suggestion) brings books to read out loud. The first one is *Black Beauty*, which I like, but not as much as I used to like *The Wind in the Willows* with Mrs Gordon. *Black Beauty* lasts a few weeks, and then Mum starts on *Little Women*.

'Mrs Gordon says her girls always liked *Little Women*,' she says.

Beth's my favourite.

The weeks fly by, and soon I'm out of bed and learning to walk all over again. This time it is even harder.

'Come on, Lucy, I won't let you fall,' says Mrs Hopkins, the physiotherapist. 'I didn't let you fall last time, did I?'

'No, but last time I could see, and it didn't seem so frightening. Now I keep thinking there's a hole in the floor in front of me and I'm going to fall down into it.' I feel really scared.

'But, Lucy, there weren't any holes in the floor last time. Why should it be any different now?'

'I don't know,' I'm trying hard not to cry, 'but it is.'

15

I'm home for the last bit of the summer holidays. Already I'm looking forward to going back to Brilbeck House. But two days before term starts, something odd happens. I've been visiting next door (this is something that Mum doesn't know I do), and as I come back down the side passage, trailing the fingers of my left hand along the brickwork, Stephen runs up to me and grabs me.

'Oh, Lucy,' he gabbles, 'Mummy and Daddy are crying in the bathroom.'

'What? Why?'

We step into the kitchen, and Rosemary runs in to join us.

'I don't know, but Daddy shouted at Rosie, then he ran upstairs, and now they're both crying,' Stephen says.

'I'm frightened,' says Rosemary, clutching my sleeve.

'What are you children doing here?' snaps Mum, coming into the kitchen. 'It's nearly time for dinner – go upstairs and wash your hands. Quick, now.'

Dinner is a strange, silent meal. It's a relief to see Jill when she arrives to take us to Sunday school. Bedtime happens without the usual games with Dad.

What's happened? Is it something that I've done?

Things remain very odd at home for the next two days, and I am pleased to get back to Brilbeck House. Although I'm in my second year now, I'm still the smallest child in the school.

Will I ever grow tall? Just a little bit taller would do. I ask my friend Alison to fill me in on everything that's happened in the months I've been away in hospital. The most important change is that Miss Wakefield has left. She and Mr Swift got married in the Easter holidays. Our new teacher is Miss Harman. I get the feeling that Miss Harman doesn't like me very much; there's something cold, perhaps wary, about the way she talks to me. Alison tells me Harman is 'difficult to please'.

And she is. Even when I get all my sums right (which, to be honest, is most of the time), Miss Harman is grudging in her comments. One day, when she picks up my Taylor frame to look at my work, she asks me, 'Why are you always so sulky?'

No one else says I'm sulky. I'm sure that I'm not. But what can I do? I mutter, 'Sorry, Miss Harman,' and bend my head over my work. But I'm thinking, This is not my problem – it's your problem, Harman. And I stop worrying about it.

But the great thing is that I am now having piano lessons. I don't know how this came about. I suspect Miss Honeybourne has pushed for it, or maybe Mr Stewart decided of his own accord.

Whatever, one Monday at dinner time Miss Harman says to me, 'At two o'clock, Lucy, you're going to Mr Perks for a piano lesson. It's been decided to see if you can manage it.'

I can tell from the tone of her voice that the decision had nothing to do with her.

Mr Perks asks if I have ever played the piano before, and I tell him about Mrs Gordon and how she showed me how to pick out one or two hymns.

'"Abide With Me" was one of them,' I tell him.

'Will you play it for me?'

Nervous, at first I stumble over the notes, but soon, as I remember Mrs Gordon and our wonderful mornings down at the River Bank, the tune flows free and sweet.

'Very nice,' says Mr Perks. 'Which hand were you using?'

'My right one.'

'Can you do it with the other one?'

'I don't know. I've never tried.'

'Have a go now.'

My fingers trip over each other, and I really stumble this time. 'Sorry, sorry.' I must get it right, or they might stop me coming.

'Don't worry.' Mr Perks takes my right hand and places my fingers on the keyboard. 'These are the black notes – do you know how they're arranged?'

'Yes. Two and then three, all the way down the piano.'

'That's right, Lucy. Now find the two black notes in the centre. The pedals will show you when you're in the middle.'

'These?'

'Very good. Now play the white note to the left of the two black ones. Excellent,' he says as the note sounds. 'That's middle C. The white note before the two black notes is always a C.'

I play all the Cs, from the bottom to the top. Then I laugh aloud with pleasure.

I can hear the smile in my teacher's voice as he says, 'The white note between the two black ones is D. So the white notes go C-D-E-F-G-A-B.'

'C-D-E-F-G-A-B,' I echo. 'What are the black notes called?'

'We'll leave them for the time being and concentrate on the white ones.'

Piano lessons are on Mondays, and every day I practise on the library piano after my Braille lesson. At first I always think of Mrs Gordon, but after a while I find the music takes me to all sorts of different places; some of them possibly not in this world.

In October I'm twelve, and Mum and Dad come all the way from home for a birthday visit. Well, they say it's for a birthday visit. But actually I think it's just an excuse: they have some news they want to tell me. Dad's got a new job. He's working as a porter in the very same hospital where Cousin Jill works. I tell them that sounds lovely. Working with Cousin Jill!

But neither of them sounds happy. They say they have something else to tell me. I wait, tightening my grip on Gwenny. The family is moving to a new house, which I shall have to learn my way around when I come home for Christmas. I don't ask why. I have learned never to expect an answer to that question.

I will discover later, from the social worker, Miss Briggs, what has happened. The house we lived in for all those years in Bridgend Lane, next to the humpbacked bridge and not far from the farm where Dad worked, was a tied cottage (Miss Briggs has to explain to me what that is), so when Dad lost his job on the farm, we lost our home as well.

At the end of term, Mum comes to collect me by train. When the train pulls into the station, there is Miss Briggs, waiting to give us a lift home in her car. It's only as we are pulling up in front of the new house – a terraced house, number eleven – that Mum tells me that Stephen and Rosemary have their own bedrooms now, so I'll be sleeping downstairs.

'It'll be easier for you,' she says.

For a moment I am speechless. Then, as the house is obviously empty, I ask where Stephen and Rosemary are.

'Jill's taken them for a walk, so that you can get settled with the house quiet.'

A whole new house to learn.

Mum positions me with my back against the closed front door. 'If you follow the left-hand wall, you'll come to the living room, where you'll be sleeping on the settee under the window. All the old things are there: the settee, the sideboard, Daddy's desk, the dining-room table and chairs, and the three-piece suite from Bridgend Lane.' I hear a catch in her voice. Oh dear, poor Mum. 'You can find where everything is in there tomorrow,' she goes on. 'Why not go back to the front door now?'

I retrace my steps.

'If you follow the right-hand wall you'll come to the stairs. There are thirteen steps,' she adds, 'and they're rather steep. You need to climb them to get to the bathroom and the toilet.'

I struggle up the stairs, counting them as I climb. Mum's right: they are very steep.

'The toilet door's there on your left. The bathroom's right in front of you.' She takes my hand and opens a door. 'Do you need to go now?'

'Yes, please, Mum.'

She ushers me in front of her into the narrow room and lifts my hand, saying, 'This is the chain.' Then she places my hand on the toilet roll holder on the wall. 'I'll wait outside,' she says, and shuts the door.

16

Mr Perks has entered me for grade one piano. I should be feeling excited, and grateful, I suppose, that Mr Perks has faith in me, but all I feel is disappointment: the day of my piano exam is the very day that Jill and Dan have chosen for their wedding. I shall have to miss the wedding, and that makes me feel sad.

January and February pass by. I practise hard every day, trying to banish my sadness by playing.

The day of the exam – and of the wedding – dawns: a bright, blustery March morning. When Miss Honeybourne asks me what I would like to wear, I choose my green pinafore dress.

'Good choice – with the primrose-yellow jumper?'

'Yes.'

I'm the last candidate before lunch, so I've got plenty of time to think about the wedding that's taking place without me. I pull myself together: I must do so well in my grade one that Mum and Dad, Jill and Dan, and Aunt Renée and Uncle Bill will be proud of me.

'You're Lucy Holland, is that right?' asks a man with a deep, quiet voice.

'Yes, sir – I'm doing grade one.'

'Good,' he says. I can hear the smile in his voice. 'There's nothing to be nervous about, I'm sure you know the pieces well. Are you ready to play the first one?'

I begin to play. At the end of the third piece I sigh with relief. I did it, I did it! Then I play scales, and then the examiner asks me to clap the rhythm of 'Three Blind Mice'. Clapping is difficult for me, but he sounds satisfied.

'Good,' he says. 'Now, beat time to this tune.'

My performance this time is not quite so good.

'Hmm, well, never mind. That's everything now – you can go and have your dinner.'

I join Alison on the window seat outside the dining room.

'How did yours go?' she asks.

'I messed up the beating time, but the pieces went all right. How about you?'

'Got a bit stuck in the second piece, but it came out all right in the end. He was nice, wasn't he?'

'Yes. I liked his voice. He sounded as though he was smiling.'

'There you are, Lucy.' It's Miss Harman, sounding a little bit warmer than usual. 'Look what's come for you.' She places a large bouquet of flowers in my lap. 'There's all kinds of spring flowers, and here's a card – shall I read it?'

> *Hope your piano exam goes well.*
> *Love and kisses from Jill, Dan, Mum and Dad.*
> *xxx*

It's too much for me. I burst into tears.

'Come on, Lucy. There's nothing to cry about. We'll put the flowers in water. They can stay in the dining room until Monday, then we'll take them down to the classroom. Come on now, dry your eyes.'

But I can't stop crying. I wanted to go to the wedding. I wanted to go so, so much. My family are all at the wedding enjoying themselves, and I'm left out. No comfort can reach the deep, dark hole inside me, but I can't say anything; I mustn't say anything, or they'll know how wicked and ungrateful I am.

17

A whole year passes, and it's summer again. I am thirteen years old, and I'm still the smallest child in the school. Out in the garden of our new home, number eleven, I am wandering deep in the American South, my fingers tracing the progress of Topsy as Miss Ophelia tries to make her behave like a girl, and less like a tomboy.

This house in Long Street was meant as temporary accommodation. Two years is a very long temporary. I know that Mum asks the council regularly if we can be given another house, and the answer always comes back that there's nothing available.

Somewhere in the background, I become aware of shoes scuffing along the edge of the pavement. Then a whisper tweaks my ear: 'There she is. The blind monkey.' The last phrase becomes clearer as their voices rise. Bolder now, they begin to chant, 'Blind monkey! Blind monkey!'

I try to pretend I can't hear, and redouble my concentration on my book. If I take no notice they'll go away.

'There you are, blind monkey!' Wild giggling, then rhythmic stamping on the pavement as the chanting resumes. They are very close to me: just a few feet away.

I'm crying now, and trying to huddle behind my book.

'Blind monkey's a crybaby! Blind monkey's a crybaby!'

Then there's a rush of feet up to me and the book is yanked from my hands. A slap, a slither and a dull thud, followed by laughter.

'Look out, someone's coming!' Feet run away down the road and around the corner.

I don't like going outside. I'm scared of them. Later Mum asks the council if we can fence off the garden to give us some privacy, and after a while, permission is given. Dad installs a fence six feet high.

How do they know when I'm out here? They must be waiting, peering through the cracks between the planks of wood, for no sooner am I settled outside with my book than the banging and the chanting start. *Bang, bang, bang* against the fence, the rattle of sticks, and the chanting begins: 'Blind monkey in a cage! Blind monkey in a cage!'

After that, I don't get out of bed. The GP says he's going to ask Mr Ryder to make a domiciliary visit. Mr Ryder looks at my hips, knees and ankles, picks me up out of bed, and makes me walk a few steps. Then he puts me back in bed, and gently pulls up the covers. He tells Mum to let me lie on the sofa during the day, and to invite friends round to visit.

'We don't have many friends round here,' says Mum.

In fact, we don't have any.

I stay in bed and I cry a lot. 'It'll never be good again, Gwenny,' I tell my doll. 'I used to believe that one morning I would open my eyes and it would all be right again, but it isn't going to happen. I know that now. I'll always be left here in the dark, in this horrid house.' Then I whisper into her ear, 'And Mum hates it too.'

Mr Ryder, Mum discovers, has written to the council. A few weeks later we are offered a different house. The new house is in Milton, near Leamington, in a quiet road called Bentham Close. It has a garden at the front and back; the back one, like the back gardens of all the neighbouring houses, is fenced in. Mr Ryder is not the only person who has been writing to the council: Miss Briggs has also been busy, and the week after we move into the new house, a large delivery van turns up. Inside it is a piano.

The new house is a piece of great good fortune, which we offset against the bad news that Mum and Dad receive some months later. Their claim for damages against Warwickshire County Council, for the negligence at Hinton Grange that resulted in my permanent blindness, has been dragging on for three years. First of all the local solicitors wouldn't take the case because of a conflict of interest, and now Mum and Dad hear from the Coventry firm; from Mr Dean to whom I gave, with such anguish, my account of what had happened to me there. He tells us that, 'due to an unfortunate oversight', the time limit for personal injury cases has expired, and the writ for damages has been declared 'null and void'.

It's during one of the school holidays around about this time that I hear David Scott Blackhall talking on the BBC about how, the year before, at the age of forty-five, he went completely blind. He talks about the initial shock and panic, the moments of disbelief, the flaring hope that it would pass, and the dull resignation to the truth that it wouldn't. I'm sitting on my own in the front parlour, and I'm transfixed by his warm, deep voice and his understanding of my own feelings. He says he learned Braille in three weeks. Goodness, I think.

I write him a letter in Braille, telling him that I've been blind for four years and my hearing's not too good either. (I don't mention my wonky bones and the difficulties I have walking.) I tell him I think he's very clever to have learned Braille in three weeks.

18

The next few years at Brilbeck House pass happily, but at the beginning of my final year there I'm feeling a bit lonely, as Alison and my other friends have already moved on.

One afternoon in early September, Mr Tapley comes up to me and asks if I would like to collaborate with him on a script for the Christmas pantomime. He wants to do *Snow White*, he says, and suggests that we write it in rhyming couplets. 'Two lines of the same length which rhyme with each other,' he explains. 'Such as: *Once a queen had a pretty stepdaughter. Jealous she was, and plotted her slaughter. Why would a mother do something like that?*'

The words come tripping off my tongue: '*Because she is jealous and running to fat?*'

Mr Tapley laughs. 'You've got the idea,' he says.

By the end of September the script is nearly done, and Mr Tapley turns his mind to the cast. He offers me the part of Snow White, but I turn it down. I know exactly what I want to be: a fairy. It is a long, long time since I first tried to be a fairy, back in the before time, when I could still see. Now another chance has come along and there's no way I'm going to miss it.

'But there aren't any fairies in *Snow White*.'

'In this one there is,' I tell him firmly. 'I'm going to be a continuity fairy, and perhaps I could double as the mirror.'

'A continuity fairy?'

'Yes: we need someone to explain to the audience what's happening when the scenes change.'

'Hmm,' says Mr Tapley. 'I think that's rather a brilliant idea.'

By the end of the second week in October, all of the parts are filled and rehearsals are under way. Snow White is being played by Maureen Turner, who has a lovely singing voice. Brenda Jones is playing the Wicked Queen, which I consider to be an excellent piece of casting. Brenda is the most spiteful girl in the school. The family mothers have been press-ganged into making costumes, and I have asked Miss Honeybourne if the continuity fairy's costume can have stars all over it.

Then disaster strikes. Hurrying to meet Miss Honeybourne after Friday morning assembly, I crash into a boy called Dennis Bowers, and fall to the floor.

Mr Stewart picks me up. 'Can you stand?' he asks.

No, I can't. My left leg is strangely bent.

I spend the afternoon with Miss Honeybourne in the X-ray department at the hospital.

'Oh, poor Lucy,' says Miss Honeybourne, holding a bowl as I vomit for the umpteenth time.

Emerging from a doorway, the radiologist says, 'Take these X-ray plates back to the clinic. They're as good as I can get.'

The curtain rings hiss along the rail as the doctor comes in. He stands at the other side of the couch from Miss Honeybourne, and says I need to see an orthopaedic specialist.

'Mr Norton visits Brilbeck House,' says Miss Honeybourne.

'Ah, I'll see if I can contact him.'

Lying on the couch between them, I'm thinking, Why don't they talk to me? It's almost as though I'm invisible. I say loudly, 'My leg hurts.'

Back at school, I go straight to the sickbay, where Mr Norton comes to see me at the beginning of the following week. He thinks that the joint in my knee has somehow got stuck in the wrong conformation, so he gives me a strong painkiller – not strong enough – and tries to manipulate it back into place, to no avail. So then he puts my leg in plaster, leaving a small hole at the back of the knee so that, he explains, he can insert a wedge, which he'll replace with a bigger one week by week. The whole process will take at least six weeks. At this news, I burst into tears. I just can't help it.

'You can still be the fairy,' says Miss Honeybourne when she visits after tea. She strokes my hand.

'An awful fairy with a leg in plaster. Everyone will laugh at me.'

'No, they won't,' says Miss Honeybourne. 'We'll make you a lovely long dress and no one will notice.'

I turn sixteen while my leg is still in plaster. I now have sessions with a speech therapist called Mrs Millsome every Wednesday afternoon. She teaches me 'The Walrus and the Carpenter'.

'Well,' asks Miss Harman one Thursday morning, 'does anyone have any news today?'

I raise my hand. 'Mrs Millsome has taught me a long poem.'

'Can you recite it to the class?'

'What, now?'

'Yes.'

I stand up, pull back my shoulders, and announce, '"The Walrus and the Carpenter", by Lewis Carroll.' My heart is thumping. I open my mouth and begin:

The sun was shining on the sea,
Shining with all his might:

He did his very best to make
The billows smooth and bright—
And this was odd, because it was
The middle of the night…

Just keep going, I think as the words flow from my mouth. Just keep going. And then it's over. I've done it. A feeling of relief and triumph sweeps through me.

'That was very good, Lucy,' says Miss Harman.

'I don't think they should've eaten the oysters,' says Maureen.

Arriving early for my session one Wednesday, I find Mrs Millsome's room empty. While I'm waiting, I lean forwards from my wheelchair and run my hand over the table to see what's there.

Oh, what's this? A squarish machine, with rows of small round things, and above them a sheet of paper coming out at the top. Ah, a typewriter! I'm going to ask Mrs Millsome if she can teach me to type.

We perform the pantomime on the last Friday of term. The plaster is off my leg, and I'm just wearing a splint. All day I feel sick with nerves. Miss Honeybourne helps me with my costume, pulling the long dress over my head and smoothing down the skirt, then fixing my long hair back with a sparkling Alice band. My hearing aid – a much smaller version of the original one – can be tucked into my bra and hidden from view.

'Here's your wand,' says Miss Honeybourne. 'It's as tall as you, and has a sparkly star at the top.'

Mr Tapley pops his head round the door. 'Wow, Lucy, you look wonderful: every inch a continuity fairy. Are you ready?'

'I think so.' I reach out with my wand and tap him on the shoulder. 'I'm nervous, though.'

'You'll be fine, won't she, Miss Honeybourne?'

'Of course,' she replies, as she makes a final adjustment to my wings.

'Ready?' whispers Mr Tapley. 'Good luck, everyone.'

The piano plays, and the choir begin: *Here we are to tell our tale...*

I lie in bed that night with the tunes still playing in my head. I'm sorry it's over now. If only Mum and Dad had been able to come. I wish they could have seen me as a fairy with a wand. I wish, I wish, I wish.

But my wishes never come true.

How I wish I could stay on at Brilbeck House for another year or two, but now I'm sixteen I'll have to leave at the end of the summer term. One May afternoon Mr Stewart drives me to Mallen Court, a residential college for typing and shorthand. With all the tutorials I've had from Mrs Millsome, I'm really quite good at typing on my Braille keyboard, and I perform well in the test, but I feel in my bones that they're not going to offer me a place.

A fortnight later, Mr Stewart calls me to his office. I know what's going to be said even before he tells me what's in the letter that he has received.

'They think you are bright enough, but they feel your many difficulties would make the course too hard for you.'

It seems I'm going to have to give up all hope of continuing my education and eventually finding work. I'll just have to go home to Mum and Dad, and if I do, the question of money will become more important than ever. While I may not be able to earn my own living (and it seems no one at all believes I'll ever be able to do that), I still need food, clothes, and a warm room in the winter.

Miss Briggs urges Mum and Dad not to give up on their legal battle: she tells them that they'll need the compensation money now more than ever. She urges them to find another firm of lawyers and sue the previous ones for letting our original case against the county council run out of time. We have to go all the way to Birmingham for this. And then, in the end, Mum and Dad are advised to accept a settlement out of court. We are offered eight hundred pounds, which will become available to me when I turn twenty-one. Eight hundred pounds. It doesn't seem very much money to make up for the fact that I have lost my sight and will never be able to see again.

19

Bentham Close, Milton, 1960. I am sixteen years old. No more school. Ever. At first, it's like being on holiday. Then comes the slow building of a new routine.

I try out the Monday afternoon Red Cross Club. When I arrive I am sat down at a table with a Mrs Brown and a Mrs Walker.

'You can call me Judy,' says Mrs Walker, who turns out to be quite a talkative woman. 'Mrs Brown doesn't talk much. She's had a stroke. What's your name, dearie?'

'I'm Lucy. Lucy Holland. What happens here?'

'We play bingo, chat and have tea. It's good to get out of the house, don't you think?'

Someone claps their hands. 'Quiet, everybody. We have a new member today, Lucy Holland. Let's all say, "Hello, Lucy."'

'Hello, Lucy,' comes a chorus. There seem to be a lot of people here.

'OK, Nan,' says Judy, 'here's your card, and your special pen.' Something slides across the table and touches my hand. 'That's your bingo card, Lucy.'

I feel a blank piece of cardboard. 'I can't read print.'

'Oh well, I'll do yours as well as mine, then.'

'Twenty-two, two little ducks. Eighty-eight, two fat ladies…'

'Mmm,' mumbles Nan, banging the table.

'Let's see your card then, Nan,' says Judy, and then she calls out, 'She's right, Mrs Leighton.'

'Well done, Nan,' Mrs Leighton says, and a sickly, overpowering perfume sweeps over me. 'You've won this beautiful bowl of hyacinths.' She claps again, and calls, 'Teatime, everyone. Now come on, chaps, put those dominoes away.'

Over a cup of tea, Judy chatters on. 'I've got a granddaughter about your age. She works in the post office, and she's just got engaged.'

'And now it's time to go home,' says Mrs Leighton. She helps me on with my coat.

'See you next Monday,' calls Judy.

Not if I can help it.

But I do return the following Monday, and I announce to Mrs Leighton that I'm going to play dominoes. Mrs Leighton doesn't think that's a good idea: dominoes are for men, she explains, as if I am a halfwit.

I tell her, 'But I can feel dominoes with my fingers, and playing bingo when you can't read the card is boring.'

Grudgingly, my plan is approved. I feel as if I have won a small victory.

'But you must return to the ladies' end of the hall for tea,' says Mrs Leighton bossily.

I smile in agreement. What does she think will happen to me over the teacups?

'Well, look what we've got here: a pretty lass.' Someone gives a low wolf whistle.

Mrs Leighton is not yet out of earshot, and swoops back. 'That's enough of that, Ben. If you're going to be naughty, I'll have to take Lucy back to the ladies' end of the room.'

'Sorry, Mrs L., just expressing my appreciation.'

The dominoes clack as they're shuffled.

'Ladies first,' says a different voice. 'Choose your seven.'

I pull seven dominoes forwards and run my fingers over the dots. 'I've got double six.'

'Lucky as well as pretty,' murmurs Ben.

'Careful, Ben,' says the second man.

It's pointless being told I'm pretty. It's not as if any man will ever want to go out with me. But I suppose it's better than being ugly, that's all.

'Can't go,' says Ben, knocking on the table. 'Your turn, Lucy – have you got a four or a six?'

'Yes, I've got double four, and I'm out.'

'Definitely a lucky one.' Ben pats my hand.

On Tuesday and Thursday mornings I have the house to myself, when Mum goes out to her cleaning jobs. For a while, until the cold creeps into my bones and makes my fingers too stiff to move, I play the piano. Then I retreat to my chair in the corner of the back room, next to the gas fire, and travel far away with the characters of whichever book I'm reading: *The Glory of Clementina Wing*, or *Marguerite's Wonderful Year*. I always choose novels with a girl's name in the title, hoping for a story of romance. Maybe I *am* pretty, but love will never happen to me; so I shall take it where I can find it: in books. Sometimes the books make me cry, sometimes they make me laugh, sometimes both. Mabel Barnes-Grundy's *Marguerite's Wonderful Year* is the funniest book I have ever read, although in the end it is sad.

Most afternoons Mum does the ironing or bakes cakes or biscuits with the wireless on in the background. I enjoy listening to *Woman's Hour*: I like the discussions, and I love the serials. The serialisation of *Mary Wakefield* sends me off in search of Mazo de la Roche's other *Jalna* novels. What joy – there are sixteen of them! In the end, I feel as if I myself am a member of the Whiteoak family.

Some afternoons, when *Woman's Hour* is over, a couple of neighbours come round for a gossip. I get terribly bored.

The women grumble about prices in the shops: 'I told him he could keep his best cuts at that price, and bought belly pork as usual,' moans Joan.

I notice that they always seem to prefer their sons to their daughters: 'Brenda's getting completely out of hand. I told her she looked like a tart in that short skirt. "You mark my words, my girl, and don't come crying to me when you get into trouble,"' says Leyla.

'They're all the same these days,' Joan remarks. 'At least my Johnnie won't be bringing babies home.'

'You're lucky, Joan,' says Mum, 'not having any girls.'

It isn't that Mum doesn't love me and Rosie, but she worries so. Especially about me. She doesn't have to worry about boys or babies, but she worries about where the money for a new coat or shoes is to come from.

One afternoon, the social security inspector pays us a visit. Mum and I sit on one side of the round table in the parlour, and the inspector sits opposite. I can hear him turning the pages of his notes.

'You've never made any one-off claims for large items?' he says.

'What kind of things?' asks Mum.

'Well, my notes show that your daughter has lots of health problems: arthritis, and bronchitis in the winter, for instance. You could claim for money to buy extra blankets to keep Lucy warm, or a winter coat or a pair of shoes, perhaps.'

Mum squeezes my hand. Then she leaves the room in a hurry, muttering about the kettle boiling over. Coming back with a tea tray, she asks, too brightly, 'Milk and sugar?' I can tell from her voice that she's been crying. 'Lucy is our girl, she's our responsibility,' she says, and rests a hand on my shoulder.

'It's not scrounging, Mrs Holland,' says the inspector sternly.

On Friday afternoons we take a bus into town and I go for a piano lesson while Mum does the weekly shop. My piano teacher is called Miriam Leyman, and she plays the organ in the church. By now I have reached grade five. I often think of Mrs Gordon, who first showed me how to pick out tunes on her piano, and who introduced me to the wide world of books and fired my love of reading.

Sunday is my favourite day. It brings in the wider world; wider, anyway, than the narrow compass of my everyday life. We have dinner and tea at the round table in the front room. Dad tells stories about the hospital where he's still working as a porter, and Stephen and Rosemary chat about their school friends and their Saturday jobs. In the evening, I go to church. There I discover that every week, on a Thursday, the minister and his wife host a gathering of young people at their home.

I am shy at first, but I'm soon made to feel welcome. One Thursday, I'm sitting at the end of the sofa, drinking a cup of tea, when the door opens and another group of young people come in.

'Lucy Locket, what are you doing here?' says a voice from the past.

'Alec? Alec Peters, is that really you?'

Turning to the rest of the room, Alec explains, 'Lucy and I were at boarding school together, a pretty grim place, a long time ago.' He tells me that his mum has recently moved to Milton, and that he's studying English at university. 'And what are you up to these days?' he asks.

'Oh, I'm just at home with my parents,' I admit, embarrassed. 'I... I'm blind, you see.'

'I know,' says Alec gently.

With Alec for company, I enjoy Thursday evenings more than ever. Sometimes a group of us go out later for a meal. I'll never forget the first time we went to the Chinese; I'd never eaten any kind of foreign food before then. I climb the stairs to the dining room between Alec and Tim, with Julie bringing up the rear, heading towards a mixture of smells I have never before experienced.

'What are you going to have?' Julie asks.

'I don't know.'

Alec says, 'I'm having curry.'

'OK, I'll have curry too.'

'Hot, miss?' asks the waiter.

'Yes, of course.' Aren't curries supposed to be hot?

'Going to try chopsticks?' teases Alec.

'No, thanks. A spoon will do.'

It smells lovely, I think as I lift the first spoonful to my mouth. 'Oh God, someone please give me something to drink.' My whole body is on fire.

Tim passes me a glass of something, which I down in one gulp. It's cider.

The rest of the curry doesn't seem so fiery. Finishing it, I think, Yes, I definitely like curry. I listen to my friends talking, laughing, arguing, and interrupting each other, while I sit silently, happier than I have been in a long time.

Leaving the restaurant, I am walking on air. I feel the heat from Alec's hand tucked under my arm. Reaching the car, he unlocks the passenger door and guides my hand to the seat. I slide onto the smooth leather. Then I lean to the right, and lay my hand for one second on the seat where I know Alec will soon be sitting.

I'm fine in the car, but at home I suddenly feel terribly sick. I just make it to the bathroom in time to throw up in the toilet.

'Well,' says Mum, who has followed me in, 'that'll teach you not to eat nasty foreign muck.'

On the contrary, I'm definitely going to try more of it.

One sunny afternoon soon afterwards, I'm wandering with Alec around the church fête when we come to Bowling for a Pig, which Julie is in charge of.

'Well, Julie,' says Alec, 'I suppose it's easier than trying to keep a wriggling pig in a pen, but don't you think a china piggy bank is a bit of a cheat?'

Laughing, Julie replies, 'I don't think many people in Milton would want a real pig in their back garden, do you?'

'You've got a point there. Anyway, show the pig to Lucy.'

'Here's its tail, and that's its nose,' Julie says, moving my hand around the money box.

'Hold on, schoolmarm,' Alec interrupts. 'She's not one of your infants, you know.'

'Sorry, I was just trying to show her.'

'How about we all go for something to eat later?' says Alec.

'Sorry, I can't. Tim and I are off to the pictures.'

As we walk away, Alec asks, 'How about you and me going for something to eat, then?'

'That would be nice,' I reply.

Now, whenever Alec is home from university, we go out – sometimes for a jaunt into the countryside, sometimes to the pictures, and we always have a meal out: Chinese, Indian, or even Turkish. On cold, wet days he comes round to our house and we stay indoors, sitting side by side on the sofa, playing chess and listening to Cliff Richard on the record player.

Season follows season, year succeeds year, and little changes. This fallow time, I will realise later, is rich with learning. If nothing else, all the books I read increase my vocabulary and widen the narrow horizons of my world, taking me beyond the confines of my cosseted existence. Stephen leaves school and gets a job. Rosemary does well in her O levels. There are always my meetings with Alec to look forward to, when he comes home to see his mum, and comes round to ours and says, 'Hey, Lucy, let's go out.' Sometimes I cry a little bit in bed before I fall asleep, although I know I shouldn't. What, really, do I have to complain about? In my dreams, I visit a country where I see flowers in bloom and the green of the trees, and I walk along sunny paths, hand in hand with Alec.

20

In October 1965, I turn twenty-one. Mum and Dad organise a party for me in the church hall, and Mum gets a friend of hers to make me a new dress: a white jersey wool dress, with a tailored look.

'New white shoes and a fancy hairdo, and you'll be the belle of the ball,' says Mum.

I open my presents after breakfast. From Mum and Dad I get a tactile watch with an elasticated metal bracelet.

'It's silver,' Mum points out, 'so it'll go well with your new white dress.'

From Stephen and Rosemary, a small brass alarm clock.

Mum taps my left index finger on each number in turn. 'Now, if you feel around, just inside the numbers, you'll find a kind of wheel with one dot on the edge. Push it round clockwise – that's how you set the alarm.' She takes the clock out of my hand and moves the dot around herself, then winds the alarm key. The alarm starts ringing.

'That's brilliant. But where are Stephen and Rosie? I want to thank them.'

'Stephen's gone fishing with a friend and Rosie's out at her Saturday job. You can thank them later.'

In the afternoon Jill comes round with a present from her and Dan: a new lipstick and powder compact. 'Open it up,' she says, 'wind the small key, and pull up the lever.'

It starts to play 'The Blue Danube'.

'Oh, it's another musical box!' Suddenly, I am taken back to a Christmas many years ago, when I could still see: the firelight, the glittering Christmas tree, and a musical box with a beautiful couple waltzing to 'The Blue Danube'.

Later, I stand by the church hall door, welcoming the guests. Uncle Bill and Aunt Renée have come over from Wales.

'Happy birthday, my favourite niece,' says Bill, giving me a big hug.

'You look lovely. Doesn't she, Bill?' says Renée.

'Beautiful, my dear,' he says, and pats me on the head.

I wish people wouldn't do that. I may be small, but I am no longer a child.

Alec arrives with Julie and Tim. 'We've clubbed together to buy you this.' Alec puts a small box in my hand.

I flip up the lid. It's a ring.

'It's adjustable,' says Julie, 'so you'll be able to get it over your knuckle.'

'There's a central black stone – jet, I think,' adds Tim.

'And it's surrounded by sparkles,' says Alec, squeezing my hand.

'It's lovely.' I put it on.

A mountain of food is laid out on trestle tables down one side of the hall: sandwiches, cheese and pineapple on sticks, slices of pork pie, sausage rolls, and glass bowls of sherry trifle. The birthday cake stands on a table of its own.

Jill takes me by the hand and leads me to the cake table. 'I'll describe the cake to you. It's beautiful. White with red icing roses around the edge, and "Happy Birthday" with musical notes all around it written in pink icing.' She traces my finger along the notes, then puts a knife into my hand and guides it as I cut the first slice.

Everyone cheers and sings 'Happy Birthday', with Uncle Bill playing the accordion.

'Now,' says Mum, 'time for games! Get into a circle, everyone.'

I find myself standing in between Rosemary and Julie. I wonder where Alec is standing. The accordion starts up again, and a large pillowslip is handed from player to player. Then the music stops and people shriek with laughter as someone pulls a garment from the pillowslip.

'Dad's got a pair of long johns,' Rosemary tells me, laughing. 'They look really silly over the trousers of his suit.'

The music begins again, then stops.

'A woman over there has got a pair of men's pyjama bottoms. She's trying to stuff her skirt into them,' shrieks Julie.

And so it goes on. I try to enter into the spirit of the game, but as I can't see the ludicrous costumes that people are wearing, I find it hard to join in the fun.

Getting ready for bed later, I pull a new nightie over my head, and then I pause. I don't want to go to sleep yet.

I start to line things up on the dressing table: to the left, my hairbrush; next to it, a bottle of sandalwood perfume. I pick that up and spray a little on my hair. In the middle, my new brass alarm clock, with its soft, steady *tick*, *tick*, *tick*. To the right, my new lipstick in its golden case: a shame to shut it up out of sight in my make-up bag. On the right-hand end of the table I carefully place the musical powder compact. I open it and wind it up: oh, to be dancing to 'The Blue Danube' with Alec! I put the ring box next to the perfume, but decide not to take the ring off. I would have liked the ring to have been from Alec alone, but that can never happen.

A few days later, Mum and I take the coach to Birmingham to collect a cheque for eight hundred pounds: the out-of-court settlement agreed by the Coventry solicitors.

'How do you do, Mrs Holland?' says the judge when we arrive. 'And this is Lucy?'

'Yes, this is our little Lucy.'

The judge pauses for a moment. 'Shall I make the cheque out to you, Mrs Holland?'

'No, it's Lucy's money.'

'But you and Mr Holland are Lucy's next of kin, and her guardians.'

'Lucy can manage her own money.'

'Well, if you're sure, I'll write out the cheque for eight hundred pounds payable to Lucy Holland.'

The following day, we have an appointment with a bank manager.

'So, young lady, you would like to open an account with this bank?'

'Yes, please.'

'Can you sign your name on this piece of paper for me, please? First, write "Lucy Holland". Now "L. Holland". Hmm… I'm afraid your signature would be easy to forge. So to protect your money and the bank's reputation, I suggest that in order to withdraw money from your account, you visit this branch in person, or sign a cheque which your mother countersigns.'

'If you think that's really necessary,' I say. I wish it didn't have to be this way. People treat me as if I am a child.

21

When Mum's out at work one day, I decide to make a pot of tea for her for when she gets back.

I start off by looking for the tea in the pantry, working my way along the first shelf: tins, jars and packets. Two large cardboard packets stand at one end of the shelf above. I take one down and put my hand inside: two paper bags, one of them open. My fingers touch something rough: Weetabix? The other box is probably Shredded Wheat. I take that one down and feel inside: yes, there's the dry feel of the pillow-shaped Shredded Wheat. Next comes a Tupperware box, where I know Mum keeps the Welsh cakes. Then the biscuit tin. I open it and help myself to a Jammie Dodger with its round of sticky jam. No cups and saucers, though, let alone the tea caddy. Stretching up, my hands hit the underside of the third shelf. The top of it is out of reach.

I leave the pantry, and slide my hand along the kitchen door until I come to the gas cooker. I examine the four rings, but no: there isn't a kettle anywhere. But what's this on the floor? A stack of open plastic racks, holding a variety of vegetables. I run my hands over the dry, earthy texture of the potatoes; the papery skin of the pungent-smelling onions; and the long, cool carrots.

Next comes a free-standing cupboard to the left of the sink. I pull out the vegetable stack and open the door, but no – only cleaning stuff: dusters, and flat, round tins of lavender polish. The drawer at the top holds cutlery, I know, plus a rolling pin and pastry cutters. Voilà – here it is: I've found the kettle at last, standing on the top of the cupboard.

But my triumph is short-lived. The kettle is switched off at the plug, and struggle as I might, I can't reach it. On the draining board, too, the drying rack for the crockery is empty. Mum must have put everything away before she left. Running my hand along the top of the work surface, I find the bread bin and the butter dish. Still no cups; just an empty glass beside the plate of sandwiches and the banana that Mum left out for my lunch. I reach up again, but can only touch the underside of the cupboards. I want to scream with frustration, 'Why, why, why me?'

After dinner the next day I ask, casual-sounding, 'Mum, where do you keep the cups and saucers? When you were out yesterday I wanted to make a pot of tea for when you came home, but I couldn't find anything.'

'What?'

Oh dear. I knew she'd get into a state.

'No, Lucy, you mustn't try things like that. Kitchens are dangerous places. You could get scalded.'

'But Miss Armstrong's blind, and she makes tea.'

'That's different, you're not like her. Things like that would be dangerous for you. Promise me not to try such a thing again.'

'OK, Mum,' I say. There's no point anyway if I can't find the cups and things. I'm not allowed to do anything interesting or exciting; nor even the ordinary things that other people do all the time. I'm fed up with being cosseted. It hardly feels like living at all.

Sometimes, in bed at night, I am an opera singer, on stage at Covent Garden; sometimes I am a concert pianist, playing Beethoven's Emperor Concerto to a packed Albert Hall; at other times I am a Liberal MP delivering my maiden speech to the

House of Commons, challenging my fellow MPs to do things to improve the lives of disabled people. Do they ever think about what handicapped people do when we leave school? Do they think about where we go; what happens to us; what kinds of lives we lead?

The months slide by, and then the years. Stephen moves into management at the factory where he works; Rosemary leaves home to train as a nurse. Then she marries and has two little boys. Except for my weekly visits to church, and the Monday evening choral society, I rarely leave the house. Occasional shopping trips with Mum, and monthly meetings with other blind people from around the county, are my only social life. The vicar and his wife have moved on, and his replacement doesn't seem interested in providing activities for young people. Singing in the choir is lovely, and I love learning the alto line of the various choral works we sing, but I don't really get to know the other members; merely saying hello and goodbye to the woman who sits next to me.

Charlotte Briggs is still an important figure in my life. She manages to secure a small, regular grant to cover heating costs for the front room, which is now where I spend most of every day, with my piano, the wireless, and my talking books, leaving Mum and Dad free to watch telly in the other room when they get back from their jobs. It's as if we're all leading separate, parallel lives.

I no longer dream of Covent Garden, or the Albert Hall, or the House of Commons. How could I ever have been so naive, so stupid?

22

One dull July afternoon in 1971, when I am twenty-six, I get up from where I'm sitting on my own in the front parlour, listening to the radio and knitting a jumper for my youngest nephew, and walk through to where I hear voices in the back room.

As I open the door I hear my mother say, 'No, there's no need to worry Lucy yet. She'll find out soon enough when the time comes for her to go and live with Jill and Dan.'

'When am I going to live with Jill and Dan, and why?' I ask.

'Not for a long, long time, darling.'

'But why would I go to live with them anyway?' My heart is thumping; my voice beginning to rise.

Charlotte Briggs speaks. 'At some time in the future, Lucy, your mother and father may not be able to care for you. We have been making plans against just such an eventuality.'

'Don't I have a say in the matter? At this rate, you'll be ordering my coffin next.' I swing around, slam the door behind me, and stumble upstairs in tears. I don't want to go and live with anyone, not even Jill and Dan. And I hate people always deciding what should be done with me. Why can't I choose for myself? Why can't I live my own life? Does the fact that I am blind make that impossible?

Over the next few weeks, on the surface, life in Bentham Close appears to go on as usual. Nothing is said about the family meeting with Charlotte Briggs; nor about my reaction. I try to appear calm, but underneath, it feels as if a pack of mice are scurrying through my brain; first one way, then another. I know what I want: a home of my own, a job like other people, an ordinary life. But how? Am I mad to think that these things might be possible?

One morning, I get a call from my friend Janet, who lives with her aunt and uncle in a house just round the corner. 'Listen, I've got some news. I'm going to do O level English at an evening class at the college.'

'That sounds interesting. I wonder if I could go too? Wouldn't it be fun to do something like that together?'

'Why don't you apply? They can't eat you.'

I duly apply, and as the days pass without a rejection I begin to allow myself to dream. I dream of sitting in an ordinary classroom with Janet; of reading, writing, and talking about books with the other students and a wonderful, sympathetic teacher. In my head, that teacher has a voice like Miss Honeybourne's.

But the letter, when it comes at last, puts paid to my foolish dreams. Mum reads it out:

> *Dear Miss Holland,*
> *I have discussed your request to join our O level English evening class with the tutor. We are unable to enrol you, as the course is held on the second floor of the college, and there is no lift. The tutor also feels unable to teach a totally blind student.*

I blink away the tears that have welled up. I hate to cry in front of my mother.

'Never mind,' says Mum cosily. 'I tell you what, I'll get Daddy's Trafford catalogue and we can choose you a new winter coat.'

'All right.' You think everything can be made better by a spot of shopping, a cup of tea or a hot meal, I think, but it's not that simple.

'Come on, Lucy, cheer up. It's not the end of the world.'

Not for you, perhaps, but I did so want to go to college. I'm always being told I can't do things. Work, love, and anything else that others do are not for people like me.

'Let's see.' Mum flips through the pages of the catalogue, wafting the scent of printer's ink in my direction. 'Here we are, ladies' winter coats. Mm, well, there's a beautiful white one with two front pockets and a neat collar, or this blue one with buttons on the sleeves. There's also a red one with a fur collar and cuffs. Which one would you like?'

'The red one sounds nice, with the fur collar and cuffs. Red's my favourite colour.'

'Sure you wouldn't like the white one? It looks like mohair.'

'No, I prefer the sound of the red one.'

'Oh well, I'll get your dad to order it when he gets home.' As she bangs shut the catalogue, another whiff of printer's ink floats by.

I wonder how Alec's getting on in his job at the publisher's? I miss him terribly since he moved south.

'Lucy, darling,' says Dad a week later, 'here's a parcel from Trafford. It must be your new coat.'

'Ooh, let's see.'

'Yes, it's definitely a coat,' he says, laying it on my lap.

I run my hands over it. 'But it hasn't got a fur collar!'

'Oh dear,' says Mum. 'They must have sent the white one by mistake. But as it's here, let's try it on.'

'But I wanted the red one.'

'I know, love, but try it on anyway.'

I stand up obediently.

'That's right…left arm first…now the other one. It looks lovely on you, doesn't it, Dad?'

You win, as usual. 'Oh well, I'd better have it, then.' There's no point in making a fuss; she'll only stop talking to me, and I hate it when she does that. And after all, she's the one who has to look at the coat. I only have to wear the blinking thing.

Part Three

1

I need to leave Bentham Close. I need to leave Mum and Dad. I need to find, and claim, a life for myself. But how on earth do I do it?

On Sundays I always listen to *In Touch*, which is regularly presented by David Scott Blackhall, the man I heard all those years ago talking about the trauma of going blind. One Sunday he opens the programme by saying, 'Today we will be talking about a new mobility technique which has just been introduced to this country from America. It is called the long cane system.'

I sit upright in my chair and listen closely as an American mobility officer whom Blackhall is interviewing says that a person with a long cane, unlike a guide dog user, can go entirely at their own pace. They move the cane in an arc in front of them, so that they always know that there is space ahead for them to move into.

'So,' says Blackhall, 'this new mobility aid would be particularly useful for elderly, frail people who walk slowly?'

'Yes, indeed,' replies his interviewee.

A little bubble of excitement moves inside me. Well, I'm not old, but I certainly can't walk fast, and they say I'm fragile, so perhaps a long cane would be the thing for me.

The next morning, I wait until Mum goes out to do the shopping, then I go into the front room and pick up the phone. The phone is a recent acquisition, and I love it. It took me no time at all to

143

learn how to use it. I put my index finger into the correct hole and begin to dial Charlotte Briggs's number, which I know off by heart.

'This is Lucy – Lucy Holland,' I say when she picks up the phone. 'I was listening to *In Touch* yesterday and they were talking about a mobility aid which has just been introduced here: the long cane. They said it can be used by elderly people who can't walk fast enough to have a guide dog, and as I can't walk very fast either I was wondering if I could have long cane training.'

'I don't know, Lucy. I haven't heard anything about this mobility aid.'

'But you'll find out?'

'I suppose I could make enquiries. I can't promise anything, mind.'

It takes three weeks for Charlotte Briggs to make her enquiries, and then to come round to Bentham Close. What she has to say is not what I was hoping for. It appears that I don't do enough walking to benefit from long cane training.

'I mean,' she says, 'you only walk around the house, don't you? When you go out shopping with your mum she pushes you in a wheelchair. Besides that, the nearest place where training is offered is the mobility centre in Birmingham, and we'd have to take you there and back every day for several weeks.'

They think I'm not worth spending the money on. Well, we'll see about that.

I know that Mum has set aside the following morning for her annual jam-making marathon. Outside the kitchen door, I listen carefully to satisfy myself that she's fully occupied. Now is the time to go for it. With extreme caution, I open the front door and step out, pulling it to behind me. I hold my breath, hoping Mum hasn't heard.

After what seems like an age, I move off in the direction of the gate. I lift the latch and step onto the pavement. Which way now? I shiver with fear. Then I turn right. I feel my way along the hedge, sliding my feet as if I'm skating, until I come to another closed gate. I'd better count the gates as I go, otherwise I won't know which is ours. After a while, the hedge gives way to a wooden fence. That's better; they're not as scratchy as hedges.

Then the fence stops and there is nothing for me to touch. Now what? There might be steps, or a hole. You never know what's just beyond your toes. Now I've got this far, though, I'm not turning back yet. Oh well, here goes. I take a deep breath and, holding my hands out in front of me, lunge forwards and almost bang into the opposite post. Wow, scary. I shuffle on past gates, hedges, fences, and occasional walls. Then nothing. This isn't like the open gate. There's grass under my feet. I gasp in fright as my hair is suddenly snagged. I raise my hands to try and free myself, but my hair is snarled up in a thorny bush.

'Can I help?' asks a stranger; a man. 'You're well and truly tangled, aren't you?' There is a laugh in his voice.

'It's not funny!'

'No. I'm sorry for laughing, but you do look odd with your ponytail and ribbon caught in the roses like that. Here, let me.'

And I'm free.

'Your hair's rather untidy, I'm afraid,' he says, patting at it, 'but I don't think you've been scratched or anything.'

I shake my head. I don't like him touching my hair. My feet find the pavement and, reaching out, my hands touch the fence. 'Thank you,' I mutter. 'I must be going now.' Not waiting for a response, I set off back the way I came, my heart thumping in my chest. I'm in a bit of a panic, but I don't forget to count the gates, and as I reach ours I shout out in triumph. 'Eighteen!' The path to the front door is easy, but how on earth am I going to get in? I have to go around the house and in through the kitchen.

I open the back door, smells of hot jam hit me, and Mum says in surprise, 'What on earth have you done to your hair, Lucy? It looks as though you've been through a hedge backwards.'

'I was trying to see if I could do the ponytail for myself.'

Mum tuts loudly. 'It's a complete mess. Get your brush and I'll sort it out before anyone sees you. I can't have people saying I don't look after you properly.'

Now, whenever I know for certain that Mum's busy in the kitchen or the back garden, I slip out of the front door and down the road. After my second trip to the corner (this time taking care to avoid the entangling roses), I decide to turn into Hume Avenue. Here too, I find hedges, fences, and more brick walls. The gates are larger on this road, and they are often open. Crossing open gaps never gets less scary, but somehow I always manage it. By the end of the second week, I've mastered Bentham Close and Hume Avenue, but I don't know what lies around the next corner.

One evening I ask casually, 'Dad, when you take the scooter round the block, what are the roads called? I know Bentham Close turns into Hume Avenue, but what's the next turning to the right called?'

'Locke Drive – that brings you to Kant Road. Then there's Pascal Crescent, and then you're back to Hume Avenue. It's possible to get all round the block without crossing any roads,' he adds.

'And where does the jitty come?'

'A little way down Pascal Crescent. Why are you so interested in our streets all of a sudden?'

'Just wondering.'

It takes me six weeks to negotiate my way around the whole block. I have even learned how to navigate the jitty, the shortcut down Pascal Crescent. It's scary, but exciting. My favourite part of the walk is Locke Drive, where halfway along there's a low wall I can sit on if I need to catch my breath. One afternoon, as I'm sitting on the wall, an ice-cream van stops and rings its chimes right in front of me. I've got a little money in my pocket, so I walk over to where the chimes are ringing and, for the first time in my life, I buy myself a large cornet. I can hardly believe how wonderful it tastes. It is the taste of freedom.

2

I won't give up on the long cane. Every Monday and Thursday morning at 9.30, I ring Charlotte Briggs's office. If she isn't there, I always leave the same message: 'I want to talk to Miss Briggs about long cane training.'

Is it my perseverance with the telephone that pays dividends; that wears her down into actually doing something about the training, or is it my perseverance with independent walking (which, as I discover, she has been told about)? Or, I will wonder some time later, was the seed sown in her mind that terrible afternoon when I walked in on them all discussing my future?

Who on earth's that? On a Tuesday morning, when everyone knows that Mum's out at work, I hear a knock at the door.

I open the door and ask, 'Who's there?', adding, 'Mum's out just now.'

'I want to talk to you, Lucy. Can I come in?'

'Oh, Charlotte – yes, of course.' And I step back into the hall.

'How about a cup of tea while we chat?'

'I can't make tea. Mum says kitchens are dangerous places for blind people. Anyway, the tea, the cups and the saucers are out of my reach.'

'I'm sure I'll be able to find everything. How about it?'

'A cup of tea would be good. Mum only leaves me a glass of cold milk.'

Once we're settled with our drinks, Charlotte says, 'Lucy, I came this morning knowing you would be alone. I have something particular I want to talk to you about. I was wondering if you would agree to go away for a while on a special course.'

'What kind of course?'

'Well, it's called a rehabilitation course. You'd be taught to cook, wash clothes, iron, shop, and clean a house.'

'But how can I go shopping if I can't go out alone?'

'The course would include some long cane training.'

'You mean I can have long cane training after all?'

'It would be hard work, and you'd be away from home for fourteen weeks.'

'I don't mind hard work. Well, I don't think I would,' I correct myself. 'But…how can I? Mum won't let me go.'

'You leave your mum to me.'

Charlotte Briggs is as good as her word. She returns the next day to talk to Mum about the advantages – to Mum herself, it seems to me when we discuss it later – of me being trained to shop, cook, iron, wash and clean. Mum agrees to discuss it with Dad on Saturday, his half-day.

But Saturday brings disaster. Mum has just gone into the kitchen, saying that she must turn down the pot of cawl that's simmering on the stove, when the phone shrills.

I pick up the receiver. 'Hello?'

It's someone from the hospital's personnel department. Dad has collapsed. He has had a heart attack.

*

The next day, in the hospital: it's strange sitting beside Dad. It's usually me in the hospital bed and others visiting.

'It's Lucy, Dad,' I say, stroking his inert hand as it lies outside the covers.

He starts fretting.

'No, Jack,' says Mum, 'you mustn't take the mask off. It's helping you to breathe. Please, darling, let it be.'

'Mm, mm,' Dad mumbles, and scratches at the mask.

'I know, love, but please leave it on,' repeats Mum.

'I really think you and Lucy should go home now, Mrs Holland,' says the ward sister. 'We're going to give Mr Holland more aspirin, and some diamorphine to ease the pain and help him to sleep. You should go home and get some rest yourselves.'

'The sister's right, Mum,' I say. 'You've been here since yesterday afternoon. Rosemary will be back soon, and it won't help Dad if you become ill too.'

The next three weeks are filled with a constant round of hospital visits. One cold afternoon in mid-February, Dad is brought home by ambulance. We all know that he will not be returning to work. Mum's Tuesday and Thursday cleaning jobs are now an even more important part of the family income, supplementing the social security payments.

Life in Bentham Close settles into a new rhythm, and time flows by almost imperceptibly. I take on the role of keeping Dad cheerful.

'Lucy, go and talk to your dad. I'm off to the shops, and he's down in the dumps again today.'

I open the back-room door and say, 'Hi, Dad, how about a game of cards? You haven't let me take any pennies off you yet this week.'

'I'm not really in the mood.'

'Come on, cheer up. Try smiling – you never know, it might bring the sun out for a change.'

We chat together for hours. He tells me all sorts of stuff that I never knew about: the workhouse where he grew up; his struggles as a young man in the '30s; the back-breaking work on the farm. I never really knew Dad before. Well, not what went on inside his head. I have an inner life that others never glimpse, but I never thought of others having one too. I suppose I always believed that they were too busy living.

3

My rehabilitation training has been forgotten, it seems. I have to stay at home to help with Dad.

Then one evening in early September, an unexpected visitor turns up. He is Mr Duncan, vice principal of Holly Bank Further Education College where Janet was doing an evening class in O level English; the place that turned me down when I applied. He explains that they are running a new English O level class – a day release class, mainly for trainee nurses and electricians – which is held on the ground floor. As there are a few places left, Mr Forbes, the tutor, has offered me a place if I can provide someone to come with me to the class as an assistant. Once he has explained all this, Mr Duncan asks if I am still interested.

'Yes, I am,' I say. I feel like shouting, 'Yes, yes, yes! You bet I am!', but I feel this may not be appropriate. I don't know who I'll get to help me, but I'll try my damnedest to get someone.

'Well then, we'll look forward to seeing you at 2pm a week on Tuesday. The class is from two to six. The first two hours is English language, then there's English literature for the second half. I'll get Mr Forbes to send you a reading list. Nice to have met you, Lucy.'

The following morning, I give Janet a ring, and she suggests that her Aunt Nancy might like to help.

'Ever since I started doing my evening class, she's been saying she'd like to do O level English too. I'm sure she can give up one afternoon a week.'

The next week, when Nancy Russell and I take our places in the front row of the classroom, a woman leans forwards and says, 'I'm glad to see you two. Last week I was the only one over sixteen – it was rather unnerving.'

'Quieten down,' says a male voice, 'and we'll do the register.' This must be Mr Forbes. 'I know you don't like it, but your employers are paying and they insist on knowing that you're here. John Wilkins, Jackie Duggan, Ann Tracey, Mrs Baines, I'm pleased that you decided to give us another go. I was afraid that last week's chaos might have frightened you away.' He pauses, then goes on. 'We have another two new members in the class today: Mrs Russell and Lucy Holland.' He hesitates for a moment. 'Lucy is blind, so she will be reading Braille – is that correct?'

I nod, feeling a strange mixture of anxiety and excitement. Under the desk I clasp my hands together, as my heart thumps. I pray that I'll be able to manage.

'Now, today I thought we'd start with a writing exercise. I'll give you a series of words and you have to write two sentences for each, showing the word's different meanings. For instance, the word "current".'

I hear the squeak of chalk on a blackboard.

'C-U-R-R-E-N-T,' spells out Mr Forbes. '"I watched a current affairs programme on the television last night", "The current in the river is very strong." Get the idea?'

I nod. The other students settle down, noisily, to write. Chairs creak, paper rustles, and some people breathe heavily.

'How will you write, Lucy?' asks Mr Forbes.

'I can do sighted writing, but not very neatly.'

'Do your best, and we'll see how we go. First word: "mean".'

Again I hear the sound of chalk on a board, and I begin to write. For the next twenty minutes I write painstakingly, conscious all the while of the sound of scratching pens, and a few mutterings from some of the others.

'Right, now, John Wilkins, you go first: your two sentences for "mean".'

John Wilkins reads out his sentences.

'Lucy Holland, can you do the last word?'

'I could only think of "A cad and a bounder."'

'No, Lucy,' says Mr Forbes, 'not "bounder". The word begins with an "F".'

'Oh.' I feel myself blushing, and I have to think quickly. 'You mean "The founder of the orphanage", or "If you go too close to those rocks, the boat will founder"?'

'Exactly,' says Mr Forbes. 'Well done. Very well done.'

In the literature class, our Shakespeare set text is *Romeo and Juliet*.

'It's a romance,' Mr Forbes tells us, 'so you youngsters should enjoy it.'

Much laughter greets this. Do I still count as a youngster at twenty-eight? I may not be as young as the rest of them, but I know I'm going to enjoy it.

Over the next couple of weeks Charlotte Briggs exerts herself to find me a reader for the O level set texts that are unavailable either in Braille or as talking books. She finds a reading service that is organised from Kenilworth; Milton lies outside their usual area, but the man who runs it, Albert Edwards, agrees to come and meet me and see if he can arrange something.

When he comes a couple of days later, I like him immediately. I tell him what I think I'm going to need. Most of the set texts – *Ten Twentieth-Century Poets*, *Far from the Madding Crowd* and *Romeo and Juliet* – are available in Braille, but Laurens van der Post's *The Lost World of the Kalahari* is not. There is also the problem of not being able to read my feedback from Mr Forbes.

'Right,' begins Mr Forbes, '*Romeo and Juliet*. We'll read it through as a class. John Wilkins, you can be Friar Laurence. Anne Jones, the nurse. Michael Johnston, you can read Romeo, and you, Lucy, can be Juliet.'

Nancy digs me in the ribs.

'But…but I can't!' My voice shakes in panic.

'You've got a Braille copy,' says Mr Forbes. 'You'll be Juliet.'

I hear half-suppressed giggles from some of the other students.

'What's funny, Derrick Barstow?' raps out Mr Forbes.

'Nothing, sir. Sorry, sir.'

'You lot in the back row can read the parts of the servants and the citizens, so pay attention. I'll begin by reading the prologue.'

I open the book. It's a good job I've read it through. I can run my finger down the left-hand margin until I come to 'JUL', and then if I move up a line I should be able to come in at the right place.

> *NURSE: Where's this girl? What, Juliet!*
> *JUL: How now, who calls?*

That wasn't too bad. Where next, though?

> *NURSE: Your mother.*

JUL: Madam, I am here. What is your will?

It's difficult to listen when I'm frantically looking for my next entrance… Gosh, the nurse goes on a bit. Wow, nearly to the bottom of the next page.

ROMEO to JUL: If I profane with my unworthiest hand
This holy shrine, the gentle sin is this:
My lips, two blushing pilgrims, ready stand
To smooth that rough touch with a tender kiss.

I wish Alec would say such things to me – in modern English, though. Careful, Lucy, you'll lose your place.

JUL: Good pilgrim, you do wrong your hand too much,
Which mannerly devotion shows in this;
For saints have hands that pilgrims' hands do touch,
And palm to palm is holy palmers' kiss.

Wow, that's quite a speech. I wonder if I can keep it up?

NURSE: Madam, your mother craves a word with you.

Oh dear – here's where Romeo finds out she's a Capulet.

ROMEO: What is her mother?
NURSE: … Her mother is the lady of the house…
I tell you, he that can lay hold of her
Shall have the chinks.

I wonder what 'chinks' means?

'That'll do for today,' says Mr Forbes. 'We'll continue next week. Not too bad. It would have been better, though, if some of you had done as I asked and read it through beforehand.'

At tea that night I say to Mum and Dad, 'You'll never guess what happened at college today.'

'What?' asks Dad.

'Mr Forbes made me read the part of Juliet in *Romeo and Juliet*.'

'That's nice,' says Mum. 'Here's your knife and fork, love.'

'Juliet!' says Dad. 'I bet you were brilliant.'

4

'I've read and marked all of your essays,' says Mr Forbes. 'Most of them weren't too bad. Some of you could do better if you tried.' He is walking around the classroom, handing out our essays. 'Anne Jones, not bad. Mrs Baines, good. Mrs Russell, interesting.'

It's the beginning of the spring term.

Mr Forbes stops in front of me, puts his papers down on the desk, and says, 'Lucy, I'd like to talk to you after class this afternoon. Please stay behind for a few minutes when the others leave.'

For the rest of the afternoon I am sick with fright. Deep down inside I know that Mr Forbes has decided that he doesn't want me in his class any longer, and he's going to throw me out.

At last I am alone with him in the classroom. Nancy Russell has gone outside to wait in the taxi.

'Lucy,' says Mr Forbes, 'where did you go to school?'

It's all too much for me, and I burst into tears. Between sobs I manage to tell him, 'I went to Brilbeck House. It's a special school for blind children with other handicaps.' Then I can't say any more.

'I thought it must be something like that. You don't realise what you've done, do you?'

'What I've done?' I manage to croak.

'Yes. The essay you handed in is A level standard. I was wondering why you're on an O level course, and, come to that, why you didn't do O levels at school?'

'Nobody did exams at Brilbeck, except for piano. Many of us never learned to read and write at all.'

'Ah, I see – but you'll certainly take this O level in June.'

'Do you really think I can? Actually take the exam?'

'Of course you must sit the exam! I am going to make enquiries about getting Braille papers for you. I suppose you could type the answers. This is your typing? The essay, I mean.'

'Oh yes, I type all of my own work.'

And so, amazingly, I sit the exam in June. A last-minute flurry from the Royal National Institute for the Blind about getting the papers Brailled in time is sorted out by Bert Edwards of the reading service – heroic Bert, as I now think of him. I barely have time to relax after the exam before I have to prepare for the fourteen-week residential course at Chester Grove. Charlotte Briggs has been busy on my behalf: she is as keen as I am for me to do the course, and is determined not to let me miss this opportunity. They are expecting me on 4 July.

Mum is, predictably, far from enthusiastic. 'Who's going to keep your dad cheerful?' she asks at least once a day.

Then, the week before I'm due to go, I overhear a conversation between Mum and Charlotte. Mum is sighing loudly.

'It's hard trying to make the money go round now Jack's not working, and now we'll lose Lucy's benefits while she's away as well.'

It makes me feel guilty, but oh, how I long to learn to live independently!

*

The reading service's annual general meeting is due to take place on the Saturday before I leave for Chester Grove. Bert has told me that the guest speaker is David Scott Blackhall from *In Touch*, and I've made plans to get back early from a day out with Janet. But the best laid schemes, as I know from Robert Burns, gang aft a-gley. On the motorway one of the tyres blows out, we have to wait for the AA, and we get back much too late for me to attend the AGM. I feel very disappointed.

The next morning, Mum shakes me awake. 'Hurry up and get dressed. David Scott Blackhall is coming round for coffee. He'll be here in ten minutes.'

Bert at work again, I think, as I get dressed as fast as I possibly can. Mum rushes away to prepare a tray of coffee and biscuits, and I get downstairs with a couple of minutes to spare before Bert arrives with David Scott Blackhall. We have a dreadfully stilted conversation about *Romeo and Juliet*; stilted on my side, that is. I feel so shy I hardly dare say anything.

'Well,' says David, 'I'm so glad we've met. At last! You sent me one of the first Braille letters I ever received.'

'When was that?' asks Mum, who has been hovering throughout.

'Oh, years ago. I think you were about thirteen, weren't you?' He pauses, then goes on. 'I'd been speaking about how difficult it was for me to come to terms with going blind. In particular, the problems associated with finding my way around.'

Suddenly, I lose my shyness. 'And now,' I say boldly, 'I'm going to be learning to use a long cane. It's something I heard about on your programme.'

'That is fantastic news,' he says. 'You must be very proud of Lucy,' he remarks to Mum.

'Yes, yes, of course,' she says.

Sometimes, though, I wonder.

As they leave, David and Bert wish me all luck for Chester Grove, and at the last minute Bert presses a leaflet into my hands and says, in a low voice, 'Get someone to read that to you soon.'

I sense that it might be something that Mum shouldn't see, so I quickly push it underneath the sofa cushion for later retrieval.

5

'I think that's everything packed now,' says Mum. 'Remember, Lucy, if it gets too hard, just ring and I'll find a way to come and bring you home.'

'Yes, OK, Mum.'

No way. I'll stick it out no matter what.

My first impression of Chester Grove is that it's a bit like Brilbeck House. Charlotte Briggs drops me off just in time for lunch, so I enter to the smell of boiled vegetables, and a soundscape of clacking cutlery, chatter, and laughter. These are familiar, and not unwelcome. But this isn't a school for children; it's a training centre for adults, and as I listen to the voices around me and start to distinguish one from another, I deduce that I am probably one of the youngest students.

The people on my lunch table are keen to tell me what they think of the place.

'I've got another six weeks to go,' says a woman who introduces herself as Lydia. 'I have learned a lot, but I wish they wouldn't treat us like kids.'

'What do you mean, like kids?' I ask.

'For example, we are all called by our Christian names, while the staff and official visitors are Mr, Mrs or Miss.'

'There are also lots of petty rules, like at a boarding school,' says another woman. 'You'll find out soon enough.'

I don't care, as long as I get my mobility training.

Later that afternoon I find myself sitting across the desk from a Mr Wells.

'Well, Lucy,' he begins, 'I'm quite worried about you and long cane training. I doubt that we've got a cane short enough, and then there's your hearing problem. Your hearing is non-directional, am I right? We'll just have to see how you manage the traffic. Then there's the worry about you and cooking. You're so small I doubt you'll be able to reach anything in the kitchen.'

My heart sinks. Why did they let me come if they were going to be like this?

Mr Wells clears his throat. 'I've allocated you to Mr Redman's mobility group. I have another concern: with you being so small and all of our trainees being visually handicapped, I'm afraid of you getting knocked over. When you walk around, make sure people know you're there: wear loud shoes, and sing or something as you walk along.'

What? Wear loud shoes? Sing as I walk?

He sighs. 'That's all for now. You'll have your first meeting with Mr Redman tomorrow morning at ten o'clock. Miss Janson is going to show you to your room so you can unpack before tea.'

Miss Janson seems both kinder and more practical. She puts my suitcase on the bed, tells me where the toilet and the bathroom are, and leaves me alone to unpack. I push the case further down the bed, and sit down beside it. Well, I'm here at last. I hope it's going to work out OK. Still, there's no point in worrying about it now. Let's get unpacked.

As I stand up, my hand knocks against a small table beside the bed. Good – I can put my tranny radio there, and the clock. I follow the wall around to the door of the room, and then on to a sliding door, behind which are some shelves. Knickers, socks and nighties here. Then another sliding door; my coat, which Miss Janson took from me, is already hanging up inside. I reach up and feel some empty hangers. Too high for me to use. Next comes a sink set into a vanity unit. On the wall above it I feel the lower edge of a mirror. No use to me. Underneath, my foot kicks a wastepaper basket, and I touch towels folded over a rail. Another corner, and I brush against a curtain and find a radiator under a windowsill, and a comfortable chair.

'Now I'm back at the bed,' I say out loud. I open the suitcase and take out my transistor and my small brass alarm clock, and put them on the bedside table, well away from the edge. I turn the radio on. It's playing the final movement of Beethoven's Sixth. I hum along to 'The Shepherds' Farewell' as I put away my clothes. Mr Wells was not exactly encouraging, but I like this room. Suddenly, I feel optimistic.

After breakfast the next morning, I'm taken to one of the craft rooms, where I meet Mr Jarvis, who sets me to making what he calls a 'trinket box'. I spend the first hour sandpapering the sharp edges of the cedarwood box, and listening to the conversations between the others.

'When did you go blind?' a woman asks.

'Eight months ago. It was quite a shock. It happened just like that, when I was doing someone's feet. I was a chiropodist.'

'Really? That must have been scary,' says a man.

'I should think the patient was pretty upset too,' says another woman.

They all laugh.

At ten o'clock the door opens and someone asks, 'Is Lucy Holland in here?'

I stand up. 'I'm Lucy.'

'Hello, Lucy, I'm Mr Redman. I've come to fetch you for your first long cane training session.'

He takes my hand and leads the way down a long corridor. At the end, he opens a door and we enter a large, echoey room.

'This is the mobility hall,' he says, shutting the door. 'Here you'll practise long cane technique, and try to walk in a straight line.' I can tell that he's smiling.

'I'm not very good at walking in straight lines.'

He laughs. 'Ah well, we'll see what we can do now, hmm?' I hear a rattling, like when Dad looks for a bean stick in the shed. 'I thought so – they're all much too long. We'll have to improvise. What about this thin walking stick?' He comes over and stands in front of me. 'Yes, almost the perfect length – the cane needs to come up to your chest bone, here.' He taps my sternum. 'Yes, good – a coat of paint, and it'll make an ideal long cane for a little person.' He puts his hands on my shoulders and lines me up against the door. 'Now, let's see you walk straight across to the wall opposite.'

'OK.' I try not to tremble. I hate open spaces, but surely he won't let me walk into something or fall down a hole; not on my first day. With my hands held out in front of me, I take a deep breath and set off. I hit the far wall sooner than I expected.

'Not bad, not bad at all. Now turn around and walk back. Yes, you drifted a bit to the right, but not too much. The sun's shining, so how about we go for a walk?'

'Outside?' I don't like the sound of that.

'Don't worry, I won't let you bump into anything, or fall. You'll be quite safe with me. It's a beautiful day, so you won't need a coat. We'll go out the back way.' He opens a door – a different one from the one we came in by – and we step out into bright sunlight. 'We'll take a stroll to the first lot of shops. I want you to hold my left arm just above the elbow, so you'll be half a step behind me as we walk along.'

I've never walked with anyone like this before.

'Let me know if I'm going too fast.'

'No, that's fine so far.'

'We're just going down a small kerb. Now up again. Good, you managed that well. We're turning right now.'

We walk a little further; then I notice that he turns right again.

'Good – you followed my body as I moved right.'

'It was easy.'

He stops and places my hand on a low wall. 'We'll sit here and have a little chat. Have you done any walking outside alone?'

'Not much. One day last year I slipped out of the house and started to find my way around the block where I live.'

'Why did you do that?'

'I asked for long cane training, but my social worker turned me down. She said I didn't walk enough. So I decided to prove that I could. I really wanted long cane training after hearing about it on *In Touch*.'

'I see.' After a short pause, Mr Redman asks, 'Is there a particular reason why you wanted to learn to use a long cane?'

I hesitate. I've never dared tell anyone this before. 'I want to become more independent. I'm not allowed to do anything at home. Mum won't even let me make a cup of tea. I want to be able to live on my own.'

'Ah. Well, here you'll learn to cook.' It sounds as if Mr Redman thinks this is the most natural thing in the world. 'And if you make good progress with the long cane, I think you should be able to use public transport: to catch buses and so on.'

Buses! The idea is so exciting that my heart misses a beat. What couldn't I do if I could use buses on my own?

Early in the afternoon I am introduced to Mrs Hallam in the kitchen, who first of all offers me a cup of tea. She fills the kettle and switches it on, and in a couple of minutes an alarming rattling noise fills the kitchen.

'What's that?'

'We put one of these in the kettle, or a saucepan,' she says, placing a small disc in my hand. 'When the water, milk or whatever comes to the boil, it jumps up and down, making a rattling sound so you know it's boiling.'

'Clever.'

'Yes, we've got lots of little tricks like that to show you. Now, have you done much cooking before?'

I shake my head. 'No, none at all. Mum says kitchens are dangerous places for blind people.' I pause. 'Especially me, because of my other disabilities and because I'm so small.'

'Well, they *can* be dangerous, of course, but we'll show you safe ways of doing things. We'll start with the basics, and next week I'll have you doing some real cooking, cleaning and laundry too.'

For Mrs Hallam the basics start with teaching me how to make a cup of tea and butter a slice of bread – a revelation to me, and a source of great satisfaction.

That Friday night, instead of listening, as I usually do, to *Today in Parliament*, I lie in bed, going over in my head all of the events of the past three days. I can't help smiling to myself as I relive my first long cane practice session in the mobility hall.

'Now, Lucy,' Mr Redman said, 'the cane's come up nicely: bright and white.'

He told me how to move the cane in an arc to the right as I stepped out with my left foot, and to the left as I stepped with my right, tapping the tip gently on the ground in front of me with each step. As before, he started me off with my back against the door and told me to walk over to the opposite wall.

'Left, right, left, right, alternating the cane and feet.'

Now I lean over and slide open the drawer of the bedside table, just to check that my very own liquid level indicator is still there. Falling asleep, I dream that I am in the kitchen pouring out cups of tea, the liquid level indicator suspended over the edge of each cup in turn and giving a small squeal as the hot tea hits the prongs. Then the scene changes, and I am tapping my way, forwards and back, across the mobility hall.

6

The following week, Mr Redman teaches me how to get to the nearest group of shops to the centre. I start by lining myself up against the back door.

'Now, walk four steps forward.'

'Like this?'

'Yes, that was good. Now find the wall on your right.'

I edge over to the right, until my cane hits the wall.

'Follow the wall to the end of the drive.'

This is easy; I like having something to follow. I count the steps out loud – 'One…seven…ten…' – and then I tap the end of the wall.

'Now you need to turn right onto the pavement,' says Mr Redman, who is close behind me. 'Here you've got a wall on the right, and a grass verge on the left. Try to walk down the middle between them until you come to a kerb. About sixteen steps for you, I should think.'

I have to concentrate really hard. I gasp as the tip of the cane taps the kerb at the end of the path, and slides off into what must be the road. I jerk myself back.

Mr Redman puts his hand on my shoulder. 'You're doing fine.'

'Was that OK?' I feel anxious.

'Yes, really, you're doing very well. Now I want you to listen, and when you think everything's clear, cross the road. It's a quiet cul-de-sac with very little traffic.'

I take a deep breath as I step down from the kerb. Reaching the far side, I climb the low step, and breathe out in relief.

'Well done   that was excellent. Now you've got two driveways, then after a while you turn right onto the pedestrian path in front of the shops.'

I set off again and come to the first driveway. 'One,' I mutter. 'Two—'

'Whoa – you've drifted into Mrs Burton's drive. I don't think she's expecting any visitors this morning.'

I stop, confused.

'See if you can find the pavement.'

I move forwards a little, find the edge of the path, turn left to follow it to the gateway, and then right and back onto the pavement.

'Very well done. Now you've only got the turning to the shops.'

Off I go again. After a few steps I move over to the right and follow the wall. Turning at the end, I go on until I find the place where we had a rest on Thursday, and sit down.

'That was so good I think you should reward yourself by buying a treat at one of the shops.'

I stand up, walk forwards, and feel my way around a bollard. Then my cane hits the line of buildings. I pause, sniff, then turn left and find the step into the greengrocer's. I push open the door and walk in.

Mr Redman, coming in behind me, says, 'The counter's on the left.'

I reach the counter and look up.

'Can I help?' a man asks. 'Would you like to buy something?'

'Do you have any peaches, please?'

'Yes, I picked up a fresh crate from the market this morning. How many would you like?'

'Two, please.' I take my purse out of my shoulder bag.

'I'll put them in a paper carrier bag for you and you can hang it over your wrist.'

During Friday's long cane session, Mr Redman tells me that he thinks I'm ready to go out to the shops alone. He wants me to do it the very next day. I just have to tell whoever is on duty that I'm going, and remember to check in when I get back.

'Are you sure I can do it?'

'Of course you can.'

That afternoon I bake a lemon drizzle cake, following the instructions on a Braille sheet Mrs Hallam hands me. I grease, weigh, pour, rub. I like the gritty feel of the cake mix between my fingers, and the sweet smells of the sugar and the butter. I forget all about the scary thing I have to do tomorrow. I'm just stirring in some caster sugar when the door opens and the matron, Miss Janson, comes in.

'Ah, there you are, Lucy. Your mum's on the phone.'

Why is Mum ringing? Has something happened to Dad? My head is so full of what I'm learning here at Chester Grove that I have quite forgotten that this is the week that the O level results are published.

So I'm surprised, and relieved, when without preamble Mum says, 'I've got your exam results. The letter came this morning. I'll read it to you. "O level English results, candidate Lucy E. M. Holland. Language: grade A. Literature: grade C."'

'That can't possibly be right. Read it again, Mum.'

Mum reads it again. It sounds exactly the same as the first time.

'But I can't have done *that* well.'

'That's what it says. You're a really clever girl. Daddy and I are very, very proud of you.'

'Thanks, Mum – I never expected to do that well. Wow, I can't believe it.'

Back in the kitchen, I sort of float through the rest of the baking session. Mrs Hallam comes back to oversee the placing of my cake in the oven, and claps her hands when I tell her my news.

'Two O levels and a lemon drizzle cake! It's marvellous!'

After breakfast on Saturday, I return to my room to clean my teeth. I think the room could do with a bit of a tidy, so I start on that. Maybe it's going to start raining; then I won't be able to go to the shops. But when I cross in front of the window I can feel the sun on my face. I go to the loo and take a long time over washing my hands. Then I pick up my cane and wander slowly down to the lounge.

'I was just beginning to wonder where you'd disappeared to,' says Mrs Hallam.

'I was tidying my room.' I pause and then tell her, 'Mr Redman said I could go to the shops alone this morning.' Oh, please say I can't go. That you don't think I'm ready for it.

'OK, off you go, then. Just let me know when you're back.' As if she doesn't care!

I set off in the direction of the back door, but stop as soon as I step outside. What if I get lost? Then I take a deep breath and step out. I'm just crossing the second driveway when I hear footsteps and a man's voice.

'Are you OK? Do you need any help?'

'No, I'm fine, thank you.' And I walk on, knowing that it's true.

At the greengrocer's, the shopkeeper asks, 'Peaches again, is it?'

'Yes, please. I brought the carrier bag back.'

'So I see.'

Having paid, I ask for directions to the sweet shop, and make my way there, two shops further down. I go in and ask, 'Which way is the counter?'

'Over here,' says a woman.

'Where's that? I've got non-directional hearing.'

'On your right. What would you like, ducky?'

'Can I have a small packet of Opal Fruits, please?'

I get back to the centre just as people are having a mid-morning coffee. I check in with Mrs Hallam, and give her the packet of Opal Fruits.

'What's this for?'

'For you, to prove I've been to the shops.'

Mrs Hallam laughs, and says she needs no proof. Then she suggests that I offer the coffee drinkers some slices of my lemon drizzle cake. They all say how delicious it is, and I don't think they're just being polite: it's all gone in a flash. There are just a few crumbs left that I squish between my fingers and swallow.

7

One morning I join the queue outside the television lounge, clutching a letter for Miss Janson to read out to me. I find it embarrassing to hear other people's post being read out. They'll hear mine too, and I don't know who it's from. All I know is, it won't be from Alec, worse luck. I sigh.

When it's my turn I discover that the letter is from Bert Edwards, who says that next weekend he's coming to a conference close by, and could he take me out on Saturday afternoon? Miss Janson says there is no reason why I shouldn't go, and she directs me to Miss Donerson, who allocates me some time on a typewriter so that I can write a reply.

'There are two typewriters in the typing room,' explains Miss Donerson when I track her down, 'but during the evenings each session is given to only one trainee. A learner might become distracted or discouraged by someone else tapping away in the same room, especially if that person is more advanced than they are. Now, let me see…' Papers rustle as she checks her list. 'Mm, there's a half-hour slot from six to half past on Wednesday evening – you could have that one. It's before one of the new trainees. He's a comparative beginner on the typewriter, and he's another two-fingered Johnnie, I'm afraid. We'll need to break him of that habit.'

I guess that the 'two-fingered Johnnie' is Harry Ansel, who arrived last Wednesday.

Late on Sunday afternoon I'm sitting with Lydia just outside the open French doors, idly listening to the radio and chatting, when footsteps hesitate in the corridor behind us.

'Are you going to listen to *In Touch*?' The voice is warm and deep. I recognise it as Harry Ansel's.

'Yes, we are.'

'Can I join you?'

'Of course – there's room on the bench,' I say, moving up and patting the space next to me.

When *In Touch* is over, Harry asks us how long we have both been at Chester Grove.

'I'm going home on Wednesday,' says Lydia.

'I've been here just over five weeks,' I say. 'I've almost learned the route to the second lot of shops.'

'Have you been blind long?' asks Lydia.

'Yes, quite long,' says Harry. 'It's eighteen years since one of my colleagues flicked the wrong switch and a machine blew up in my face while I was dismantling it.'

'That sounds nasty,' says Lydia.

'It was. I lost the sight in one eye straight away. The other retina detached a few years later. The doctor thought it was probably loosened at the time of the accident.'

'I've got a detached retina too,' I say. 'Mine came off at boarding school when I was nine.'

'I've got macular degeneration,' Lydia tells us. 'It's been going for a while, but it took a dive for the worse about ten months ago.'

On Wednesday evening, at six o'clock prompt, I'm waiting outside the typewriter room. I write a quick letter to Bert to say I'd love to see him, and then, as I've still got time, I decide to write to Mum and Dad. I stop typing when I hear the door open.

'Sorry, do you mind if I just finish the envelope? Then I'll be out of your way.'

'No trouble,' says Harry. 'You won't disturb me.'

The address typed, I take the envelope from the machine, fold the letter and slide it in. I stop as I pass the other desk, and say to Harry, 'Thanks for that – it was good of you to let me finish. I was writing to my parents. I've never done that before.'

'Where do they live?'

'A place called Milton, near Leamington. I live with them there. You're from London, I think?'

'How do you know that?'

'Partly your accent, but I also heard you tell someone that you live down the road from Lambeth. I mustn't interrupt your typing practice any longer, though, or I'll be in Miss Donerson's bad books.'

Harry laughs, and asks me how I am going to spend the rest of the evening. I tell him that I'm going to listen to a Proms concert in my room.

'Oh, me too,' he says, 'when I've finished here.'

Saturday is a fine, sunny day, and I have a wonderful time with Bert. First we go on the river, and as the boat moves slowly upstream Bert questions me closely on what I've been learning at Chester Grove.

'You look so much more confident,' he says. 'Just in these few weeks.' He is full of congratulations on the O levels, and wants to know what I'm going to do at the end of this course, when I return home.

'Some more O levels. If I can do English, why not history, maths and so on? Although by then I'll have missed the beginning of term, but…'

'But what?'

I don't want to say more. It is all too tentative, too unsure. Perhaps I could start looking for a place of my own? is what I'm thinking.

As we're coming back downstream, a young man comes and slumps down noisily on the bench opposite us, and suddenly leans over and snatches up my hand. 'You're a pretty girl. Will you be nice to me?'

I can smell the beer on his breath, and I try to withdraw my hand, but his grip tightens.

'I think you should let go of Lucy's hand,' says Bert.

'Lucy…what a pretty name for a lovely girl.'

'Let go at once,' says Bert.

A member of the crew comes over, and just then the boat docks. 'Come along, sonny,' says the crew member, 'let go of the young woman,' and he prises the man's fingers away from my hand. 'Sorry, miss, I think he's a little unwell.'

'Five o'clock already,' says Bert when we're on dry land again. 'I don't know about you, but I could do with a cup of tea and something to eat.'

I readily agree. My right knee is giving me some gyp – it's been troubling me for a week or two now – and I never say no to a cup of tea.

We walk down the high street.

'Too late for tea, and too early for dinner,' Bert says in a regretful tone.

What is he up to? There's something behind all of this. I don't believe he is just being kind.

'That looks like a nice café, but it's empty,' he says, trying the door handle. The door swings open, emitting a ping.

'We're closed,' says a woman emerging from somewhere at the back.

'Oh dear,' says Bert, 'but Lucy and I are tired and thirsty. Do you think we could just have some bread and butter and a pot of tea, please?'

To my surprise, the woman takes pity on us, and offers to make us a ham salad. And when Bert tells her that blind people find salads very difficult to manage, she promptly offers us a Spanish omelette.

'That would be very kind of you,' says Bert.

When it comes it is utterly delicious, and for a while we eat in silence.

Then Bert clears his throat and says, 'Lucy, if you're going to pick off one O level a year, it will take you forever to get anywhere. Why not go to college and do it properly?' He pours us another cup of tea each, and then goes on. 'Did you read that pamphlet I gave you just before you came away?'

'Yes – I got Miss Janson to read it to me.'

'What did you think? Would you like to go to Wake College?'

So that's what this is all about. 'Well, yes, of course. It sounds amazing. They seem to cater for students with a wide range of physical disabilities, but the brochure didn't say anything about blind students. They are hardly going to want to have me.'

'I know the principal,' says Bert, and I can't stop a smile from chasing across my lips. Of course Bert knows the principal. Bert knows everybody! 'If you're interested, I think I could arrange an interview for you.'

8

On the way back to my room, I meet Harry in the corridor.

'Did you have a good afternoon?' he asks.

'Yes, it was fun.'

He asks me what I am off to do, and when I say I'm going to listen to the Proms, he suggests taking his radio down to the mobility hall, so that we can listen together. What a nice idea, I think.

I drop my bag off in my room, and hurry down to the mobility hall. 'Are you there?' I ask, as I push open the door.

'Yes,' says Harry. 'I've found an electric socket over here, right next to a settee.'

'Where?'

'About ten feet in front of you, slightly to the left.' He pats the sofa, and adds with a chuckle, 'Come and sit next to Uncle Harry.'

Already halfway across the room, I stop dead. 'Damn it, you're not my uncle,' I snap.

There's a shocked silence; then, in a low voice he says, 'I'm sorry, I didn't mean to patronise you.'

Reaching the sofa, I sit down beside him. 'No, *I'm* sorry. I must be a bit tired. We walked around rather a lot this afternoon.'

Harry says nothing, but fleetingly touches the back of my hand, as if to say sorry again.

We are just enjoying the end of the first movement of the Eroica Symphony when the door is flung open and two people come in. They completely ignore us, go over to the pianola and, with a great deal of laughter and shouting, put on some boogie-woogie.

'This is no good,' I say. 'There are some chairs in the corridor outside the principal's office. Why don't we take the radio down there?'

'I haven't got any batteries.'

'I'll go and fetch mine. I've got plenty of battery power.'

Later, drifting off to sleep, I think about Harry. He is really, really nice.

My dreams are a jumble of the day's events, with three phrases weaving in and out: 'Will you be nice to me? What a pretty name for a lovely girl' and 'Damn it, you're not my uncle.' The boat and the smell of the river…a Spanish omelette…and could I really go to college?

On Sunday evening Harry and I gravitate to the chairs opposite the principal's office. We haven't agreed to do so, but somehow it just happens.

'Why are you both sitting there?' asks the principal when he sees us.

'It's the only place, apart from our rooms, where we can listen to the Proms in peace,' I tell him.

'You know the rule,' adds Harry, 'about no girls in men's rooms and vice versa.'

The following evening finds us ensconced in the principal's office. 'I don't use it in the evening,' he's told Harry. 'Why don't you and Lucy take a radio down there and listen to the Proms? Anyone else who wants to can join you.'

But, though the offer is made to everyone, no one else wants to listen to the Proms.

We also meet up in the typing room. The first time, I linger to talk for a few minutes before leaving him to his typing practice. The second, he arrives well before his own slot starts, and soon after that he is opening the door to slip inside just after I arrive. We chat, and if footsteps approach down the corridor, Harry taps away on the other typewriter.

A couple of weeks pass like this, and then I'm due to cook my first proper meal, to which I get to invite a friend. I invite Harry. On the menu is cauliflower cheese, followed by mandarin jelly soufflé. Afterwards we do the washing-up together.

Then Harry has to go for his mobility lesson. 'Can I come again?' he asks.

'Perhaps.' But of course he can.

Five minutes later, just when I'm putting away the last few things, I suddenly feel very sick. I make a dash for the cloakroom, brushing past Mrs Hallam, and reach it just in time. I'm retching violently into the sink when I hear Mrs Hallam's dismayed tones.

'Oh no, that looks like blood.'

In no time at all, I find myself in the doctor's office with Miss Janson the matron, who has been called by Mrs Hallam.

'Now, young lady, I hear you've been limping, and now vomiting,' the doctor says. 'Where does it hurt?'

'My right knee's a bit painful sometimes when I walk.'

Supporting my leg, he bends the knee several times. 'Mm, it's certainly scrunching a lot.'

'I can make all my joints do that. Would you like a demonstration?'

'I think I'll forgo that one. So, Miss Janson, Lucy was vomiting up blood?'

'Yes – the domestic science tutor followed her into the cloakroom.'

'I see. What medication is she on?'

Miss Janson empties my bag of medication onto the doctor's desk. He picks up the bottles one by one.

'For a start, you can pour this lot down the drain. I should think your stomach lining is torn to shreds. Now, young woman, I think we'll put a plaster cast on your leg to give the knee a rest, and see if that does any good. In the meantime, I recommend you stay off it.'

'But what about my mobility training? I was just about to learn to use buses.'

'The buses will wait, don't you worry.' He pats my shoulder. 'After a few weeks you'll be back walking as good as new.'

It won't work. It never has before, so I don't see why it will this time. But I say nothing. And I can't even produce a polite smile.

9

The next morning finds me once again sitting across the desk from Mr Wells.

'Perhaps you should go home for now. You could come back and finish your training once your leg has healed and your stomach is better.'

'Please, please don't send me home like this. If you do, my mum will never let me come back. Please, please don't send me home.'

'Well, I'll have to talk to the rest of the staff and see what they think.' He pauses. 'Are you sure you wouldn't be better off going home to recover and coming back later?'

'No, please let me stay.' If they send me home, I'll never see Harry again.

I am allowed to stay.

I'm sitting outside in the early September sunshine, reading a book, when footsteps approach.

'I've brought you a present.'

'Why? It's not my birthday.'

'I've just been to buy some oranges, and the greengrocer asked me if the small young woman was all right. When I looked surprised, he said you were a regular customer – and a lover of peaches. I told him about your plaster and bought you two peaches: one for today, and one for tomorrow.' He places a paper bag on my lap.

He asks how I am managing without all the pills I've been taking, and I tell him that although the pain's gone through the roof, I seem to have woken up.

'It's as though a black cloud has been lifted from my brain, flooding the world with colour.'

'But the pain?'

'It's more bearable if I'm doing something. So I need to keep busy. Reading in particular is good: it's as though losing myself in a story diverts part of my mind away from the pain. It's still there, but it's a nagging background ache rather than screaming for attention at the front of my mind.'

That evening, in the principal's office, I am perched on the desk, my plastered leg supported by my wheelchair. Harry sits in the principal's swivel seat. He reaches for my hand. John Lill is playing Beethoven's Piano Concerto No. 1. As the first movement flows to a close I feel Harry's left arm circling my waist. He leans towards me and kisses me on the mouth.

'Oh,' I breathe. I lean into the kiss, returning his embrace.

That night, lying in bed, I am in turmoil. What's wrong with me? I love Alec, I've loved him for years, but now… Perhaps I don't know what love is? Or perhaps I'm a bad person? I know you can't love two people. It's not right. Thoughts chase each other round and round my head, while tears leak from the corners of my eyes and soon my pillow is damp. What am I going to do? Eventually, I fall into a troubled sleep.

*

The next morning, I give myself a firm telling-off as I wash my face. 'Try to behave like a sensible young woman,' I say out loud, sternly.

Church after breakfast, and then I spend the afternoon knitting in my room.

'I need to finish this shawl,' I tell Miss Donerson. 'My friend Becky's baby is due soon, and if I'm not careful it won't be ready in time.'

That evening I go to the principal's office as usual to listen to a concert, but 'I'm a bit tired,' I tell Harry, 'so I'll stay in my wheelchair.'

When the music begins, Harry reaches for my hand. I feel confused, and withdraw my hand from his.

Monday evening is the same. On Tuesday I slip away to my room, spread Becky's baby's shawl out on the bed, and start to knit the border. On Wednesday, Harry follows me into the typing room and sits down next to me.

'Don't you want to see me any more?'

Immediately, I burst into tears. 'No, no, it's not that.'

'What, then? You've been different since I kissed you on Saturday.'

'It's difficult.' I blow my nose. 'You see, I've been in love with someone else for years. Someone at home, called Alec… Or perhaps I don't know what love really is, and now…' I sob. 'Perhaps I'm not very nice – a bad person with no morals, I mean.'

Footsteps approach down the corridor, and Harry leans over and taps away on my keyboard until they fade. Then he gives a low laugh. 'Is that all?'

'It's not funny,' I protest between sobs.

'No,' he says, 'I know it's not funny.' He gives me a quick hug. 'No, it's not funny, but listen to me, darling.' He takes both of my hands in his. 'It's possible, in a lifetime, to love more than one person. I loved my wife Amy. You know that. After she died I thought I would go on for the rest of my life not loving anyone else, but then I met you. You can love more than one person at a time, darling Lucy. But I believe you can only run one successful relationship. So…' He pauses. 'So you are going to have to choose.'

I withdraw my hands, blow my nose again, and wipe my eyes. 'I'll have to choose?'

'Yes – I'm sorry, my love. I know what I feel and what I want, but this has to be your decision.' He walks over to the other desk and begins to type.

Lying in bed that evening, I feel more peaceful than I have for days. I'm not wicked, anyway – that's good – but to choose…

Throughout the next day, as I'm cooking, sewing or doing craftwork, my mind is miles away. I must choose… I have to decide… My thoughts go round and round without finding a way through the confusion.

In the early hours of Friday morning I wake and sit upright in my bed. There isn't a choice. All these years I've ached, longing for Alec to kiss me, but nothing. Well, not quite nothing. There was that occasion when he began to stroke my hair, and I smiled, encouraging him. Then he stopped and withdrew his hand as though he'd been burned. After that I didn't see him for ten days, and when he returned, we played chess as though nothing had happened. And two months later, he moved south to take up his job at the publisher's. Alec doesn't love me, and he never will. We will never have that kind of relationship.

I lie down. I know what I'm going to do.

*

On Friday evening, with a concert playing on the radio, I reach for Harry's hand and murmur his name. There is no need to say any more. His arms come around me, and soon we are kissing.

'Are you sure?' he asks, holding me close.

'Yes, I'm sure. In the end, there wasn't a choice. There is only you.' I kiss him once more.

With only two weeks to go before the fourteen-week course comes to an end, I receive a phone call from Bert Edwards to say that the principal of Wake College has agreed to give me an interview.

'Bert Edwards has imagination,' says Harry thoughtfully, when I tell him what Bert has arranged.

But what now for Harry and me? Now that I have made my choice, now that I have admitted to myself – and to Harry – that I want him, need him, am in love with him, how can I be parted from him?

To my shock and surprise, the day before I'm due to leave, Harry insists that we don't contact each other for the next two months; in fact, not until Christmas. 'I'm over twice your age, and a recent widower,' he says in explanation, 'and you need time to decide whether you're sure about your feelings.'

'But I love you.'

'And I love you.'

'Oh, Harry!' Suddenly I feel desolate.

10

Home seems both familiar and strange. Familiar in the pleasure of seeing Dad and spending time with him: the games of Monopoly and dominoes, and his wanting to hear about everything I've learned at Chester Grove; and familiar in Mum's litany of anxieties and complaints. But it's strange too because I feel that my life has changed, and yet I must keep quiet about that.

Mum insists on accompanying me to my interview at Wake College, having made her feelings known on my first evening at home. 'I'm not sure it's such a good idea. After all, you've already gone lame after being away from home for a while. Dr Metcalfe agrees with me. She says your place is here with us.'

Dr Metcalfe? I have always felt a coolness, if not hostility, emanating from the family GP; sometimes I wonder if my disabilities frighten her.

I've got an appointment with my old orthopaedic surgeon, Mr Ryder, the day before the interview, and Mum tries it out on him too, but he is having none of it. He gives me an injection of hydrocortisone in the joint beneath my kneecap, so painful it makes me gasp and tear up, and then when Mum starts with her complaint he tells her politely, 'Going to college would be good for Lucy. Even if she goes lame again, I would just give her another injection. No, Mrs Holland, I don't think you should worry. Lucy is a tough little being. We both know that.'

*

I feel really nervous when we arrive at Wake College. What if they don't like me? I can't say anything with Mum here, though. She's bound to suggest that we turn around and go straight home.

The day is packed with interviews – not just with the principal, Mr Lockhead, but with other teachers and staff members, and the college doctor. Mr Lockhead tells me that the college has never accepted a blind student before, and that it would be an experiment for them.

'What would you like to study?' he asks.

'History and maths O level, and perhaps A level English?'

'You could certainly do history. I'm not so sure about maths, though – none of our tutors know Braille – but we do teach A level English. In addition, all of our students do art to improve manual dexterity, and domestic science to gain independent living skills.'

'I did some cooking on a rehabilitation course where I also learned to use a long cane.'

'You are older than most of our students, most of whom are between sixteen and eighteen. Would that worry you?'

'I don't see why it should. Most of the trainees at the rehab centre were a lot older than me, and that didn't bother me at all.' In fact, I fell in love with one of them.

Next I meet Mr Longbourne, the English teacher. He is interested in discussing the practicalities around accessing books, and I tell him about Bert Edwards's reading service, which would cover for any texts not available in Braille. Then I go on to Miss Partridge, history and sociology, whom I like very much.

At lunchtime I meet up with Mum in the dining room. She has, meanwhile, been shown around the girls' hostel. I can tell at once that she is no more favourably inclined towards Wake College than she was earlier: now she's obsessing that I'm going to get knocked over by one of the wheelchair users.

After lunch I go to see Dr Bramley. At first he seems unsympathetic.

'So, you want to come and study here?' he asks.

'Yes. Yes, I do.'

'How old are you?'

'Just twenty-nine.'

'How old were you when you left school?'

'Seventeen.'

'And what have you been doing since then?'

'Not much until this year.' I clasp my hands in my lap, and go on. 'I took O level English at a college in Leamington this summer.'

'Mm. So you've wasted eleven years of your life.'

It wasn't my fault.

'If you get a place here, I hope you would work hard?'

'Of course, I wouldn't waste this chance. I really wouldn't.'

'Well,' he says, and now I can hear him smiling, 'you look strong enough. No puff of wind is going to blow you away.'

I think he likes me.

He gets me to squeeze his hands, one after the other, as hard as I can. Then he asks me to stand up and try to push him over, and says that he'll do the same to me. I take a deep breath and bend my whole weight into the shove.

'That's fine. I wanted to make sure that you wouldn't get knocked over too easily.'

By the end of the day, I am exhausted. We are told that we'll hear the college's decision at the beginning of next week. Before anything, County Hall will have to be contacted, Mr Lockhead explains, and the question of fees sorted out. Oh dear. Mum doesn't like the sound of that. She doesn't speak to me all the way home.

How I long to tell Harry about today; to hear his voice echo my hopes and allay my fears. But an agreement has been reached. I mustn't break it.

11

The next week comes and goes. And the next. Mum misses no opportunity to tell me how much Dad missed me while I was away at Chester Grove, and how no one else has my knack of cheering him up. The fact that money has been tighter than usual does not go unremarked either. One afternoon Mum casually lets drop that she's missed a number of meetings of her beloved Welsh Society, as she couldn't get anyone in to sit with Dad.

'Surely Stephen could have stayed home one evening?' I ask.

'He works so hard, he needs his evenings out with his mates.'

One evening every couple of weeks is surely not too much to ask. But Mum's always been soft on Stephen.

Finally, at the very end of the second week, there's a phone call. It's someone from the County Hall education department: they have agreed to pay my tuition fees at Wake College for two years, and my residential fees for the first year only. There will be no allowance for living expenses or books. If I wish to accept the place I must be there by two o'clock on Sunday, or it will be allocated to someone else.

'This Sunday, in two days' time?' This seems astonishing.

'Yes – the students will be returning after the half-term break.'

'Thank you,' I stammer, and put down the phone. I pick it up again almost immediately and dial Bert's number. When he answers I blurt out what County Hall have just said, and then I burst into tears. 'But I can't… I w-won't be able to go.'

'Why ever not?'

'Mum…' And I dissolve into sobs.

Bert arrives in Bentham Close within half an hour. By then Mum is in a foul mood. It's as if she knows what's going to happen. She bangs the tea tray down on the table between us.

'Your father's not well this evening, and I need to go and sit with him,' she announces, and stalks out of the room.

Bert pours out the tea and asks me to tell him what the problem is.

'Mum says she can't manage without me to help her look after Dad. Then there's the money: my social security payment is a real help to them.' I feel as if I'm choking on the words. 'I can't abandon them.'

Bert speaks fast and urgently. 'Lucy, you have got to listen to me. What I am going to say will sound cruel, but it is true. One, you do not owe your parents a living, and two, if you let this opportunity slip, you might never get another.'

'I really, really want to go to college, but I feel so selfish and guilty.'

'It's your decision, but think carefully.'

Slowly, I drink my tea, trying to calm the tumult in my brain. I take a deep breath and declare, 'I'm going to college.'

'I'm sure that's the right choice,' says Bert. 'I could drive you there if that would help.'

'Please – and would you mind coming into the other room with me while I tell them?'

Together we go into the living room.

'I'm sorry, Mum, but I'm going to college on Sunday. I can't let this chance pass me by.'

'It's not enough notice, Lucy. I can't possibly get all your things ready by Sunday. It just can't be done.'

'I've got enough clean clothes to take with me. The rest will have to come later. Bert says he'll pick me up and drive me there. Dad, perhaps you would like to come along for the ride and see the college?'

12

I sit on the bed in my hostel room. Dad, Mum and Bert have just left. I feel very alone. I'm not sure I want to stay after all. If I'm quick, I can catch them before they leave… No, don't be silly, you can't give up now. Tears are beginning to run down my cheeks. I'm really, really scared. What if Mum's right and I can't cope?

But an hour or so later I realise I am coping just fine. A second-year student called Fern has taken me under her wing.

'New places are always a bit confusing,' she reassures me, 'but you'll soon get used to things round here.'

In the evening I sit down and write to Harry. I beg him to ring me when he gets home from Chester Grove in a fortnight's time. 'I know it's against our agreement,' I write, 'but I can't wait until Christmas to talk to you. Really, I can't.'

The college has arranged for a mobility officer to come and give me a few sessions so that I'll be able to find my way around independently; I realise that some considerable thought has gone into my needs as a blind student. On the whole the other students are very welcoming, and Fern is wonderfully helpful. But there are a lot of strangers to cope with, new voices to recognise, lifts and corridors to negotiate, and work to be knuckling down to: O level history, O level sociology (both with nice Miss Partridge) and A level English with rather scary Mr Longbourne.

I am so relieved when I find out that the reader allocated to me by Bert Edwards's reading service is my old church friend Tim. He provides a reassuringly familiar voice in a noisy whirlpool of new sensation. Tim is the second still point in my turning world; the first is that, once again, I can take up the piano, and Shirley Dyson, with whom I have a lesson every Wednesday afternoon, says I can start working towards my grade five.

13

Monty Davison, the mobility officer, soon has me on the buses, as I proudly tell Harry in one of our phone calls. Our agreement not to be in touch with each other has been thrown to the winds, and now we speak regularly. We have a method: I dial his number and let the phone ring twice, then put the handset down, and Harry rings me back at once. One evening he tells me that a friend of his called Jean is planning a trip to Coventry to see some friends, and that she and her boyfriend Tony will give him a lift to Wake College. The trip is planned for the last Sunday in November or the first in December.

But he comes earlier than that. I am in the dining room and have just finished a bowl of apple crumble with yogurt when the door opens and two sets of footsteps approach the table.

'Here she is,' says a stranger's voice.

A hand rests on my shoulder, and simultaneously another voice, deep and warm, says, 'Lucy!'

'Harry!' I jump up and hug him. 'Oh, Harry, you didn't say you were coming today.'

'I didn't want to risk disappointing you.'

'Well, Harry, I'll pick you up around six. Is that OK?' says the stranger.

'Lucy?' asks Harry.

'Wonderful!' I check my watch. 'That's four whole hours together. Let's go down to my room, then we can hug each other properly.'

I hang on to his hand as I lead the way out of the dining room; I can't quite believe that he's not just going to suddenly disappear. We pause in the cloakroom while I put on my coat, and then, with Harry's hand on my shoulder, I lead the way down to the hostel and my room. Once inside, I lock the door and draw the curtains.

'At least we'll have some privacy now.'

As though on cue, there comes a tap at the door.

'Who is it?'

'It's me, Fern. I wondered if you wanted to come up to see the film?'

'Not today, thanks, I'm busy.'

'OK, see you later.' Her footsteps retreat.

We sit on the edge of the bed, clasped in each other's arms, and kiss.

'Darling Lucy,' Harry says, 'I've dreamed of this moment, and feared it would never come, and now here you are, in my arms.'

'It's been too long – much too long,' I breathe. After a while, I say, 'Harry, I'm going to have to tell my parents about you, but I'm not sure how to do it.'

'Yes, I've been thinking about that too. We can't put it off any longer if we're going to see each other often.'

I make us both a cup of coffee as we decide what our next steps should be.

'I think I need to talk to my mum. I could go home this coming weekend and tell her then.'

'Yes.' He hesitates. 'And I could write to her. That might help, mightn't it? What about your dad?'

'That's tricky. He's always poorly these days, and I don't want to make things worse by upsetting him in any way.'

As Harry puts his hand out, he knocks the mug of coffee that I'm holding.

'Oh no!'

'You're not burned?'

'No, but my dress is soaked.' I take it off and sit down next to him on the bed in my petticoat.

He slips his arms around me, and holding each other close, we start kissing again. Soon we are lying together on the bed, arms around each other.

'I do love you so,' I murmur against his chest.

'And I love you,' he says, stroking my hair.

14

'Your turn, Lucy,' says Dad.

I'm home for the weekend. I feel weighed down by the conversation ahead: the one I'll have to have with Mum about Harry. I shake the dice cup.

'It's a five,' says Dad. 'One, two, three, four, five.' He moves my Scottie dog along the board. 'Collect a card from the community chest.' He picks up a card and reads, '"Get out of jail free."'

'Ha,' I laugh. 'That'll be useful.'

'How are your studies going?' Dad asks as he shakes the cup. 'Three – I've landed on Park Lane. I think I'll buy a hotel.'

'Wow, you're doing well. I've only got two houses on Old Kent Road.'

'Your studies?'

'Fine: I've been getting good marks – mostly As and Bs – for my essays.' I hesitate for a moment. Should I tell him this, or not? 'In fact, the other day one of the lads complained that I always get good marks – better ones than he does. It's awkward. You see, Miss Partridge hands back our essays in class, and always reads out my mark for me as I can't read it myself. Because I get good marks, some of the others – the lads in particular – are a bit resentful. They call me "swot" and "teacher's pet".'

'Don't let it get to you, Lucy. They're only jealous.' Dad moves his boot around the board. 'Just go on doing your best. I always knew you were the clever one.' He pats my hand. 'You're better than I ever was at schoolwork – except for arithmetic, I always did well at sums.'

'I've always been good at sums too. I must've inherited it from you.'

I wish, I wish I could phone Harry, but it's too risky. What if Mum picks up the extension?

'Goodnight, darling,' I whisper into my pillow that night, and it gives me some kind of comfort, just as whispering to Baby used to do when I was a little girl.

All the next morning Mum's busy around the house and in the kitchen, and I can't pluck up the courage to interrupt her. In the afternoon, I've just settled down to play the piano when she comes in.

'Your father's watching the wrestling so I thought we could have a good gossip,' she says cheerily.

A good gossip! My heart lurches in alarm. When she offers me a Welsh cake I reach for it with relief.

She asks one or two questions about college. 'You're not overdoing the walking, are you?'

'No, Mum – don't fuss, I'm perfectly OK. I'm going into town on the bus by myself too these days.'

'I don't think that's a good idea. What if you fall over, or get lost? No, it's not a good idea.'

Oh dear. That was stupid of me, but hey, here goes: 'Mum, I'm seeing someone I met at Chester Grove.'

This is met with silence. How unlike Mum. Then in a very cold and slow voice she says, 'I know. He sent me a disgusting letter, which I tore up and threw in the dustbin.'

What? What is she talking about? There was nothing disgusting about that letter.

'I'm not your little Lucy any more. Next birthday I'm going to be thirty.'

'But, Lucy, I've told you that that kind of thing isn't possible for you.'

Here we go…

'And,' Mum's voice seems to thicken with outrage, 'he's in his sixties too.'

'You'd have the same reaction whatever age he was. Oh, Mum, why can't you see that I'm grown up?'

'*And* he's been married before.'

'Well, you should see that as a good thing.'

Mum makes a noise of disgust; an exaggerated retching sound. 'I'm sorry, darling, but this has to stop right now.'

'I'm not going to do that, Mum.'

'You must – I insist. And you're not to talk to your father about this. He'd only worry.'

For the rest of the weekend Mum speaks to me only when it's absolutely necessary. No more Welsh cakes. No more invitations to gossip. I feel such relief when I'm picked up on Sunday to go back to college. But I already know that Mum's reaction has only made me more determined.

As soon as I get in, I ring Harry. 'I'm not giving you up. You don't want me to, do you?'

'No, but, oh, darling, I wish it didn't have to be like this.'

'So do I, but that's Mum's choice. Now, tell me how much you love me.'

'That's impossible. There are no words to tell you how much I love you. If I was there with you, I would cover you in kisses and hold you close to my heart.'

A few days later my friend Fern asks me if I'm looking forward to Christmas, and I tell her that, yes, I always look forward to Christmas, but this year I'm not actually looking forward to going home for it. Of course, she asks why not, and I tell her.

'My mum's sent me to Coventry for having a boyfriend.'

'You're joking?' says Fern. 'You mean she won't speak to you?'

'More or less. She only speaks to me to give instructions: "Come and have your dinner!" or "It's time you were in bed." That kind of thing. No small talk or chit-chat. But I've got plenty of homework to keep me busy. And it's only three weeks.'

'That seems like a long time to me,' says Fern.

I think of all the weeks, months and years I've spent waiting while nothing happens and life goes on for everyone else, and I'm surprised by the passion in my voice when I say, 'But, Fern, it's not, not really.' And I tell her what I haven't told anyone else: that I'm going to go and stay with Harry in his flat in London for one weekend in January.

'Good for you,' says Fern.

On Christmas Eve, Alec, who's back from London to spend Christmas with his mum, takes me to midnight Mass. It's lovely, and I keep the conversation firmly on Christmas and all things Christmassy. At some point I am going to have to tell him about Harry, but right now the problem of Mum is as much as I can cope with.

When I come downstairs on Christmas morning I go into the kitchen and say cheerfully, 'Happy Christmas, Mum,' and hold out the present I have wrapped for her.

'Shh, don't make so much noise,' says Mum, ignoring the proffered gift. 'Your father's having a lie-in, he's under the weather this morning.'

'Oh dear, what's wrong?'

'I think he may have the flu.'

'I'll pop in and wish him a happy Christmas.'

'Come and have your breakfast first. I don't want dirty dishes hanging about all morning. I've got the dinner to cook.'

I do my best to cheer her up, reminding her that Rosemary and the kids will brighten things up for Dad, and that Renée and Bill are coming too. But my attempts fall on stony ground.

'It all makes more work for me,' she complains. 'And Stephen's not going to be here. He's having dinner at his friend's parents' house. I don't see why people can't stay in their own homes on Christmas Day instead of making more work for others. Hurry up, and don't keep me hanging around.'

I make one last effort. 'Oh, Mum, Harry's given me this St Christopher for Christmas, but I can't reach to fasten it round my neck. Please will you do it for me?'

'Certainly not – you've got a much better one upstairs, a gold one. That one looks like cheap silver gilt.'

Tears prickle my eyes, and I leave the room and go into the bedroom to see Dad and wish him a happy Christmas. He says he'll be up for dinner; he's only staying in bed because Mum insisted. I wonder briefly whether maybe she's forcing him to be ill so as to make me feel bad. Oh dear, how difficult she is sometimes. Oh well! What can I do? I hand over my present.

'Can I open it now?' asks Dad.

'Of course.'

'A new stamp album – and what's this?' he asks, opening an envelope and taking out a piece of paper. 'My goodness, it's a year's subscription to the Philatelic Society.'

'I thought you ought to have a society to belong to, like Mum has the Welsh Society. I found out that a member of the local group lives in Bentham Close, and he's willing to give you a lift to the meetings.'

'Lucy, you are a very kind girl.'

I pick up his hand and kiss it. 'And you are a very kind dad.'

Then I go round the corner to Janet's house for coffee. As soon as I get there, and once I've struggled out of my parka, I ask her if she'll fasten Harry's St Christopher around my neck for me. She asks if I've spoken to him yet, and I tell her no, and that it's really awkward as I don't want Dad to get drawn into the argument and get upset.

'Ring him from here, then,' she says promptly.

'Do you think your uncle and aunt would mind?'

'Of course not – I'll tell them it's a friend of yours from college.'

As soon as Harry picks up the phone, I blurt out, 'Happy Christmas, darling. I love the St Christopher. Janet's just fastened it for me.' I am so happy to hear his voice; his deep, comforting voice.

'You can't love it as much as I love the tape you gave me,' he says. 'I've been playing the carols all morning. It's heavenly having your voice here with me in the flat.'

'Oh, Harry,' I sigh, at exactly the same moment as he says, 'Oh, Lucy.'

We both laugh, and my heart lightens. I think everything is going to be all right.

'Aunty Lucy,' Rosemary's son Simon says, 'I like your necklace.' His little fingers flutter gently at my throat.

'Yes, it's lovely, isn't it? A good friend gave it to me.'

'Come on, Simon, eat up all your carrots,' says Mum. 'They'll help you see in the dark.'

'Aunty Lucy loves carrots, but she can't see at all,' replies Simon.

Everyone laughs.

'You've got a sharp one there,' says Uncle Bill.

'Well, that's the last of them gone now,' says Mum, shutting the front door after seeing Bill and Renée out. 'I'm whacked. I think I'll go to bed early straight after the news. You too, Jack – you're still far from well. I'll have to keep an eye on that cough. I think I'll call the doctor if you're still coughing after Boxing Day.'

I don't say anything. I know that this fussing is for my benefit.

'Don't fuss, Mary, I'm not that bad,' says Dad. When Mum goes out to the kitchen to make bedtime drinks, he says quietly, 'What's got into her now? Something's going on, but I've no idea what it is.'

I feel really torn. I've promised Mum that I won't mention Harry, but I think it's wrong to keep Dad in the dark like this. 'When Mum's in one of these moods it's best to leave it alone,' I say finally.

And so the holidays wear on: chilly silence from Mum, secret phone calls to Harry from Janet's house, and quiet afternoons playing board games with Dad. When it's time to leave I promise him I'll come back soon, and hope that by then I'll be able to talk openly to him about Harry.

15

A couple of weeks after I get back to college my big toe begins to hurt, and once again I am referred to Mr Ryder. By the time I see him the toe is inflamed and extremely painful.

Just like old times, Mr Ryder makes me walk across the room, and then he says, 'I think you're banging your foot down too hard when you walk. Let's try putting a bar on the bottom of your shoes to see if that helps.'

For some reason the orthopaedic shoes are sent to Bentham Close rather than to college, and when I get them, forwarded on by Mum, I find a note twisted inside one of the toes. I ask Fern to read it out to me. She smooths it out and reads it.

'It says, "Don't come home for the weekend: we won't be there." I think it's your mum's writing.'

I feel sick. 'Thanks,' I say. 'I'd better take the shoes to show Mrs Hargreaves, to make sure they're OK.'

I set off for the physio's room, but halfway down the corridor, tears gush from my eyes. Unable to hold them in any longer, I begin to sob.

'What on earth's the matter, Lucy? Here, come and sit down. Now, tell me what's wrong.'

I can't speak, so I hand Mrs Hargreaves the note.

She reads it and says, 'But I don't understand.'

'Mum's cast me out.'

On the last Friday in January I take the coach to London, and from Victoria coach station I take a taxi to Patton House in Clapham Road in Stockwell. The kindly taxi driver takes me up to the third floor and along the balcony to number thirty-two, where he rings the bell. Soon Harry and I are in each other's arms. We cling to each other.

'Oh, Harry,' I gasp. 'Oh, Harry, I made it at last.'

Ten minutes later, we are sitting on the sofa, hand in hand, when the phone suddenly begins to shrill.

'Bother,' says Harry. He steps across the room, picks up the receiver and begins, 'Stock—'

'I demand to talk to my daughter!' shrieks Mum.

'She's not here.'

'Liar! Put her on right now!'

'Not unless you calm down and behave reasonably.'

'How dare you tell me how to behave? You're disgusting, taking advantage of a poor little girl like Lucy.'

From the other side of the lounge I can hear every word. Harry doesn't have to put up with this. I cross the room and take the phone out of his hand. 'Mum, you've no right to talk to Harry like that. What do you want?'

'He's a liar. He said you weren't there.'

'I'm not surprised when you're shrieking like that!'

'You're as disgusting as he is. You're…you're nothing but a harlot, a whore. Your father's in intensive care: he's had another heart attack. If he dies, you'll be to blame. It'll all be your fault.'

How can my mother speak like this? Does she think that Harry and I are actually sleeping together? She can't think much of me if that's what she imagines. I know that he's going to give up his bed to me and sleep on the sofa tonight, but my mother has made me feel so upset and jangled, and I'm so worried about

Dad, that I don't want to go to bed on my own. In the end Harry persuades me to get into his bed, and he lies down beside me, outside the covers, and early in the morning I finally cry myself to sleep in his arms.

We don't talk much on Saturday, but we sit together quietly on the sofa, listening to music. How is Dad? How is Dad? But I'm not going to ring Mum to find out.

Sunday morning is more cheerful. We listen to *The Archers* as Harry records the omnibus.

'How long have you been doing that?' I ask as he slips the tapes into a postal wallet.

'So many years I've lost count. I send them to a blind woman called Eileen who moved to America a long time ago. It's a link with home for her.'

Then we walk to Harry's friend Jean's house for lunch, which is lovely, and then it's time for me to return to college. Harry comes with me in the taxi to put me on the coach. I don't feel as brave as I did on Friday.

'Oh, love,' says Harry, 'don't let it get to you.'

'No, I'll be fine. I just need to find out how Dad is.'

'What are you going to do?'

'I'll ring Stephen at work in the morning.'

Stephen sounds cold on the phone. He tells me that Dad has been moved out of intensive care. 'No thanks to you, though,' he says, and hangs up.

Over the following ten days I try to bury myself in work, and not to think about what's going on at home. On Thursday my sister Rosemary calls from a phone box to tell me that Dad is home from hospital. I long to talk to him, but I can't risk Mum picking up the phone.

'I want to take a look at that toe and see if the inflammation has gone down now that you've got your new shoes,' says Dr Bramley.

I take off my shoe and stocking, and lift my foot.

'Good – that looks much more normal,' he says. 'And now that I've seen to your foot, tell me what's going on at home.'

I am so surprised that I burst into tears. 'Mum… Mum's cross – *very* cross – with me, because I have a boyfriend. I went to see him in London, and Dad… Dad had a heart attack. His second one!'

'Mm, I thought it must be something like that. I hear you've been bursting into tears all over the place, and you are doing well in your studies, so it had to be something wrong at home.' He pauses, then asks, 'How long have you known this man?'

'Since last August.'

'Where did you meet?'

'We were both on a rehabilitation course in Nottingham.'

'I see. You say your mum disapproves?'

'Yes.'

'What about your father?'

'Mum wouldn't let me tell him. Then he found out, and found out that I'd gone to spend the weekend with Harry in his flat.'

'Mm. How old are you?'

'Thirty.'

'Well, I think you are old enough and, from what I've seen, sensible enough to make such decisions for yourself. I met your mother when you were interviewed here. If I remember correctly, she was very protective of you. Overprotective, I guess. Half-term is coming up soon – take my advice and don't go home. Is there somewhere else you could stay?'

'Yes: a friend in Gosport keeps asking me to visit.'

'There you are, then. I've met people like your mum before.' He pauses, and in the quiet I can hear the rain beating on the ground outside. Then Dr Bramley goes on. 'In the beginning they care for their disabled child because they love them. In time, though, they become dependent on them, subconsciously seeing them as an insurance policy against a lonely old age. If you want this new relationship to succeed, you're going to have to be very strong. In the end your mother will see that her choice is between keeping you on your own terms, or losing you altogether.'

16

At the end of half-term Harry and I are together again in his Stockwell flat, sitting on the sofa with our arms around each other.

'Are you comfortable being here alone with me?' he asks, suddenly and puzzlingly.

'What a silly question. Of course I am.'

'Are you sure you wouldn't rather have a boyfriend nearer your own age?'

'The only boyfriend I want has his arm around me right now. What's age got to do with anything?'

He catches my hand, and begins kissing my fingers. 'Love you, love you,' he says, kissing my palm.

A shiver of pleasure runs through me. 'Oh, Harry.' I kiss him again.

'I haven't got much,' Harry says. 'No savings or anything like that.'

Now what's he on about? 'I don't know what money has got to do with anything either. All I know is that I love you.'

'Your family…they are so against us.'

'That's their problem, not mine. Anyway, they don't know you, so they're not in a position to make a rational decision on the matter.' Where on earth is this conversation going?

'And you're just beginning your studies. Later, you could go anywhere, do anything.'

'It wouldn't be the same without you.'

He slides off the sofa, at the same time slipping an arm around my waist. I smile to myself. So that's what this is all about. I'm not helping you this time, though.

'Oh, I can't bear this any longer,' says Harry. 'Please, please, Lucy, will you marry me?'

'Of course I will.' I lean forwards and kiss him on the mouth.

'But you'll still be young when I die.'

'In that case, let's make the most of the time we have. There's nothing the matter with you, and surely we can count on you reaching threescore years and ten: your allotted time. That gives us ten years.' I kiss him again. 'Ten years with you will be better than a lifetime with anyone else.'

We agree that I'll write to my parents to announce our engagement, and post the letter just before I go back to college. Once that's done, Harry will let his sister Lily know, and his two brothers.

17

The next morning we walk to a jewellery shop that Harry knows in Lambeth, to buy me an engagement ring.

I know exactly what I want: a dark green tourmaline. Because of the size and weight of the one I choose, the stone has a tendency to swing around to the underside of my finger; the jeweller tries to stabilise it by fitting a ring guard, but then I can't get it to go over my knuckle. I have to laugh.

'It must make it look like a wedding ring when it swings round,' I say, 'with the gold band showing on top. But still, it's the best ring ever.'

Later on, we're talking about *In Touch* – I ask Harry to record it for me as I won't get back to college in time for it – and it turns out that my fiancé is actually a friend of David Scott Blackhall. When I tell Harry that David came to my house once (and that I was completely tongue-tied), he urges me to give him a ring and tell him about our engagement. He gives me the number and I tentatively dial it, and then I tell David that I have just become engaged to a friend of his called Harry Ansel.

He crows with delight. 'Harry Ansel! You're a very lucky girl, if you don't mind my saying! Harry is one of the nicest people I know.'

It's lovely to hear someone speak so enthusiastically about my Harry, and for it to be David Scott Blackhall is just amazing.

It cheers me up as I sit down that afternoon to write the difficult letter I must write: the one to Mum and Dad to tell them that I'm engaged to be married. It helps, too, that Harry puts on his tape of Beethoven's first piano concerto, which has become our very special music.

The following morning, when Harry's sister Lily arrives with the shopping, he tells her our news. She congratulates us both, hugs me, and says how lovely it will be to have me as a sister-in-law. I feel a warm glow inside.

So far, so brilliant. But it's Bentham Close that is preying on my mind. That afternoon I ask Jean, who's giving us a lift to the coach station, to stop the car by a postbox so that I can post my letter. I need to be safely back at Wake College by the time my parents get it. Jean stops the car and offers to jump out to post the letter for me, but I need to do it myself. I slide the envelope into the slot and, with a strange sensation in my stomach, listen to the rustle as it lands. Back in the car, I squeeze Harry's hand and lay my head against his shoulder.

News of my engagement ring travels around the college in a flash. A stream of visitors comes to my room, and I find myself stopped in the corridors by staff as well as by my fellow students. Everyone is so pleased and excited for me that I find it hard to stop smiling. The domestic science teacher, Miss Winter, suggests that I make my own wedding cake. I can't think of anything nicer.

Although I'd like to hear from Dad, I'm not really in any hurry to hear from Mum. From the silence, I suspect she is sulking. Then on the third evening after I get back, just after Tim has been reading to me (he is full of congratulations at my news), I am called to the phone. I guess it must be Mum, and I pick it up with some trepidation.

'Hello.'

'Hello, Lucy, it's Dr Metcalfe here. Your family doctor.'

'Dr Metcalfe?' Why on earth is Dr Metcalfe ringing me? 'There's nothing wrong at home, is there?'

'Wrong? I should think there is! Your mother came to see me this morning. She had just got your letter, and was very distressed.' Dr Metcalfe speaks hurriedly, in a hard, cold voice. 'It wasn't a very nice letter. You're not a very dutiful daughter, and,' she raises her voice and enunciates clearly, 'in the circumstances you're also a cheat.'

I have begun to tremble. 'How do you mean, a cheat?'

'Well, you won't be able to carry out your conjugal duties.'

'How dare you?' I shout, and then I hang up.

I am terrified and shaken by what that woman has said. I go to lectures, I read what I'm meant to read, I even manage to write a couple of essays, but all the while the phrase echoes in my head: conjugal duties…conjugal duties…conjugal duties. It begins to sound hideous to me, but I can't block it out. Is it true that Harry and I won't be able to make love? Why should that be the case? I don't really understand, but I feel a deep, dark, painful anxiety. It wouldn't be fair to Harry to marry him without being able to make love properly, so perhaps we won't be able to get married after all. I can't bear to think about it, yet I can't stop thinking about it. If anyone asks me, 'What's wrong?', I just say, 'I can't talk about it,' and hurry on. Worst of all are the daily calls to Harry. He realises that something is up, but all I say is that I'm very, very busy and I can't talk for long. I hear the concern in his voice, but what can I do? I can't tell him what that horrible woman said to me.

In the end, I book an appointment with Dr Bramley. I feel terribly embarrassed, but I have to know the truth. My voice trembles as I repeat, word for word, what Dr Metcalfe said. Dr Bramley's first reaction is anger: Dr Metcalfe is completely out of order, he tells me, and her phone call was totally unethical. I am *his* patient, not hers. Then he asks me what I know about sexual intercourse, and when I tell him – not very much, in a nutshell – he huffs and puffs and then explains the mechanics in some detail.

'I can't see any reason why you both shouldn't be able to manage that,' he says.

But then I tell him that that's not all. That I've never had a period, and that I remember that once – I must have been about thirteen or fourteen – Mum told me that the doctors had said that I would probably never have periods ('But that doesn't matter as you're never going to get married,' she said), and it has never been mentioned since. And now I feel terribly confused, and stupid.

'You should have been given the facts long ago,' says Dr Bramley gently. 'I thought this kind of ignorance was confined to the past.' He tells me that lots of women don't have periods, for one reason or another, and that it doesn't stop them getting married. 'And it doesn't stop them having full sexual intercourse,' he adds. Then he pats my shoulder and says, 'Now, let me see you smile.'

I smile. 'Will that do?'

'Splendidly!'

18

At last Dad rings up, and invites me to please bring Harry to Bentham Close so that he and Mum can meet him. I do wonder what's been going on behind the scenes, but it's only some time later that I discover – from Rosemary – that Mum 'went ballistic' (Rosemary's words) and wanted to apply to get some kind of court order to stop the marriage from going ahead. Dad had to take a firm line: he forbade Mum to do any such thing, and he told them all – Mum, Stephen and Rosemary – that I was old enough and wise enough to make my own choices.

Kind Mrs Hargreaves, the college physiotherapist, drives me home to Bentham Close on the Friday evening, and promises to collect Harry and me on Sunday at five. Harry is due to arrive by train on the Saturday morning. Dad tells me that Charlotte Briggs has offered to drive Mum and me to the station to meet him.

An inspection committee, I think, but to Dad I say, 'That's good.'

'He sounded awfully posh on the phone,' says Dad. 'I do hope this weekend goes all right.'

'You'll like him, Dad. He's really, really nice, trust me.'

Saturday goes well. Harry is enthusiastic about the egg and chips Mum produces for dinner ('Egg and chips on Saturday': I realise that she needs to show Harry that she's not putting on anything fancy for him), and helps her with the washing-up afterwards. Later, he and I play pontoon with Dad.

On Sunday morning the two of us go to church with my old friends Julie and Janet, and I introduce Harry to the Reverend Laurence Denton. Later on, Harry whispers to me that he thinks Mum went through his suitcase before we all went to bed last night. Of course she did; I feel myself blushing with the shame of it. How could she? And why isn't Stephen at home? Mum says something about 'a fishing competition' – but a fishing competition that takes up the whole weekend? I feel a bit sad. Stephen and I used to be so close when we were little. But Rosemary brings the children round for Sunday dinner after church, and that cheers me up.

'Who's he?' asks six-year-old Simon.

'My name's Harry. I'm a friend of your Aunty Lucy's.'

'Are your eyes broken like Aunty Lucy's?'

'Yes.'

'Eat up your dinner and don't ask so many questions,' says Mum, 'otherwise you won't get any pudding, and it's ice cream with rhubarb tart today.'

'If you're a friend of Aunty Lucy's,' Simon says, 'will I get more presents at Christmas?'

'Simon,' says Rosemary, 'that's enough.'

'But I want to know.'

'That depends on whether you're a good boy,' says Harry.

'You wag that tongue of yours too much,' says Mum. 'One of these days, the cat'll get it.'

Rosemary admires my ring. 'I've never seen a stone that colour before,' she says. 'I think it's lovely.'

I tell her that it's a tourmaline. She asks about the wedding, and I say that we're planning on next July, when I've finished at college.

'We needn't talk about that yet,' says Mum loudly, clattering the dishes as she clears them away.

A couple of days after I go back to college, I am summoned to the principal's office. Naturally, I think I must have transgressed in some way, but as soon as I go in Mr Lockhead tells me not to look so scared, and says he wants to talk about my work – 'Your excellent work,' he adds hastily. He says that there's been a staff discussion, and the consensus is that I should stay on at college for an extra year, and apply to go to university.

University? What? I tell him that no one in my family has ever been to university, and on top of that I don't want to wait two years to get married.

He pooh-poohs the first reason, and then says, 'Why wait at all? You could get married in the summer and come back next year as a day student. You're quite a bit older than most of our students, so I don't think it would be setting a precedent. And...' After a short pause he adds, 'It would also fit in with the county's decision to pay only your tuition fees for your second year.'

I am still struggling with the concept. 'Are...are you sure I'm clever enough to go to university?'

'If your work keeps up the way it has done so far, I have no doubt that you'll meet the entry requirements. Why not go away and think about it?'

I walk down to the hostel in a daze, with the word 'university' bouncing around in my head. I can hardly believe it. And we'd be able to get married this summer. I pass my door without stopping, turn into the telephone lounge and dial Harry's number, letting it ring three or four times.

'Harry,' I leap in as soon as he picks up the receiver, 'the principal sent for me, and you'll never guess what he said.'

'What? You sound really excited.'

'He wants me to stay for an extra year and apply to go to university, and when I said I don't want to wait two years to get married he said, "Why not get married this summer, and come back next year as a day student?"'

'I always knew you were a clever girl.'

'Yes, but we can get married this summer,' I repeat. 'Won't that be wonderful?'

'Yes, of course, darling, but what will your mother say?'

'The sooner it happens, the sooner she'll get used to the idea. Of course, it will mean you moving to Coventry. How do you feel about that?'

'As long as we're together, anywhere is fine with me.' He pauses, then says, 'I'll enquire about swapping my flat for one in Coventry. I think local authorities allow residents to do that.'

'Oh, darling, it'll be wonderful to have a home of our own.'

19

In the domestic science room one Tuesday morning, Miss Winter says, 'Well, Lucy, if the wedding's going to be this summer and you want to make the cake, we had better get cracking.'

'That's the plan, anyway,' I say. Putting on my overall, I take off my ring and slip it into the pocket. 'The date hasn't been fixed yet, though.'

'What kind of cake did you have in mind?'

'A traditional fruit cake with marzipan and royal icing. Could it be square with two tiers?'

'I think that should be doable. I'll make a list of ingredients, then you can go shopping later in the week, but today I thought you could cook a chicken curry. I told Dave, Mohammed and Jo, who are baking rolls and rhubarb crumble, that they could watch you cry as you chop the onions.'

We'll see about that, I think. I use my liquid level indicator to measure a pint of boiling stock; then Miss Winter gives me an onion to chop.

'Have you ever used a chopping bell?' she asks.

'No.'

'Well, here's one. You place the halves of the onion under the bell, then press down the handle.'

I try, but nothing happens.

'You need to bang it down quite hard.'

'Like this?' I thump my right palm down on the handle.

'Yes – if you lift the bell now, you'll find that the onion's in pieces.'

It's clever, and a lot quicker than the way I was taught at Chester Grove. Safer finger-wise, too. And no crying, either. I cut the chicken breasts into small pieces with scissors – much safer than a knife – and toss them in flour.

Miss Winter reads out the rest of the recipe: '"Fry the chopped onion in hot butter in a deep-frying pan." This one should be big enough.' She hands me a pan. '"Next add a tablespoon of mild curry powder and stir. Add the seasoned chicken pieces and keep turning until lightly browned, about two to three minutes."'

I love the smell of the cooking onions and chicken, and the sound of it all sizzling.

When everything has been simmering together for forty-five minutes, the timer pings and Miss Winter says, '"Now add a tablespoon of mango chutney and two tablespoons of marmalade, and cook for another ten minutes." And, Dave, Mohammed and Jo, as you were denied the sight of Lucy's tears, I think you ought to be compensated by helping her to eat her chicken curry.'

'And perhaps we could have your rhubarb crumble for afters?' I suggest.

Afterwards, we help each other to clear the table, wash up, and put everything away tidily. Then I hang up my overall and slide my hand into the pocket to take out my ring.

'Oh no!'

'What's the matter?' asks Jo.

'My ring!'

After five minutes' frantic search, the ring is found on the floor beneath the hanging aprons.

'Here it is,' says Jo, putting it into my hand. 'It's beautiful,' she adds, 'but I'll never have one. No one will ever want to marry me.'

'I used to think that,' I tell her, 'and now look at me: about to go and buy the ingredients to bake my very own wedding cake.'

Then comes the ordeal of going out with Mum to look for a wedding dress.

'We have to be careful not to draw attention to Lucy's deformities' is Mum's opening line to the assistant in the first shop we visit.

Fortunately, Julie, who's going to be my bridesmaid, is there to give moral support. I try on lace and satin, silk and seed pearls. They're all lovely dresses – I can feel how lovely they are, and how beautifully the material falls – but they are all much too long.

'Could the skirt not be shortened?' asks Julie, when I try on the silk.

'If we make it shorter, it won't flow,' says the assistant with authority.

In the second bridal shop we go to, the assistant also bemoans my stature: 'The trouble is, you're two inches shorter than all our gowns. And chopping off the bottom isn't going to work: they'd look odd.'

I am beginning to feel pretty disheartened. I mean, it's not as if I'm able to do anything about the fact that I'm tiny. I can't grow just to please them.

And the shoes: 'A court shoe with not too narrow a heel is best for my daughter,' states Mum.

I know she is right, but... Back in my room at college that afternoon, I have a private weep. It's not fair – all I wanted was a white wedding dress. Nothing fancy; just a dress like any other bride's. I'm fed up of never being able to buy clothes without a fuss. I dry my eyes, go to the wardrobe, pull back the curtain and take down my purple evening gown. I stroke the material and smile to myself; then, having made up my mind, I put the dress back on the hanger and go to the telephone lounge, where I dial the number of Molly Hexham, the woman who made me the evening gown.

Later, I ring home. 'Hi, Mum, I've sorted the wedding dress problem. Molly Hexham is going to make it for me. I wondered if you'd like to go with her to pick the material. I know you'll both choose something really special.'

'Well, if you're sure. Molly has made you some lovely dresses in the past.' Then she adds, 'It'll be cheaper too.'

The following week, I make my wedding cake under Miss Winter's supervision. I measure and sift and beat and fold, preparing the mixture for the two baking tins. But I can't quite manage to stir in all the fruit: the mixture is simply too stiff.

'How about if I commandeer some big lads?' suggests Miss Winter. 'I can hear Dave and Mohammed in the corridor.'

I nod my permission.

Opening the door, Miss Winter calls, 'Dave, Mohammed, come and lend us your strong arms to stir Lucy's wedding cake.'

Laughing, the two lads, followed by Jo, push their wheelchairs into the room. Taking turns, they wield the wooden spoon.

'Thanks, lads,' I say. 'I'll save you both a piece of cake.'

Guiding my hands as I slide the two tins into the oven, Miss Winter says, 'Now we just need to turn the temperature down a tiny bit every half-hour for the next three hours or so. After that, you can test to see if they're done.'

For the rest of the day the scent of slowly cooking rich fruit cake permeates the classrooms and the corridors. I am on cloud nine.

So much to discuss. So much to decide. So much to plan. The guest list: I flatly refuse to invite Dr Metcalfe, and with bad grace and considerable muttering, Mum accepts my decision. But I must have Charlotte Briggs, Bert Edwards, Alec and all of my old friends from church. We plan the reception, including, belatedly, a photographer. Neither I nor Harry has even thought about photographs until now.

'They're not a priority when you're blind,' I explain to Dad.

We have conversations with the Reverend Denton, who will be marrying us. 'I'm a bit worried about the logistics of two blind people walking back down the aisle together,' he admits.

I reassure him. 'Julie, the bridesmaid, will make sure we don't stray.'

Music: choir and organ, and at the end, a recording of our favourite music. Hymns: 'Lead Us, Heavenly Father, Lead Us' is one of my favourites, and because I've never liked the 'Wedding March', we decide we'll come down the aisle to that hymn. 'Abide With Me' will conjure up the presence of Mrs Gordon; we lost touch with her years ago, but I still think of her a lot. Our ushers will be Alec and Tim. I would like Dad to give me away, but I know he is nervous about it, and I don't want to force him. Honeymoon: we both fancy Shropshire; a hotel or guest house with full board. A lot of places refuse our booking when they discover that we are both blind, but eventually we find The Old Rectory, who say they will be very happy to accommodate us. It sounds wonderful.

Now we just need to find somewhere to live and everything will be perfect.

20

I have just got out of the bath on the morning of my wedding day, and gone through into my bedroom. I am listening to the radio with half an ear.

'Good morning on this beautiful August Saturday. The sun is shining for all the brides and grooms out there.' And then, 'Especially for Lucy Holland and Harry Ansel, who are getting married in Leamington this afternoon. Uncle Bill and Aunt Renée wish you all the best, and have asked me to play "Congratulations".' The presenter sings along with Cliff Richard for the first lines of the song.

The hairdresser is coming to the house to do my hair, and Mum's and Julie's. I have mine swept up and pinned behind, with ringlets cascading down my back. It feels fabulous. Then Julie and Jill do my make-up and nail varnish, and help me on with my dress, zipping it up and fastening my cuffs. On my head I wear a simple veil beneath a wreath of orange blossom.

I reach the top of the stairs just as the front door opens, and Uncle Bill and Aunt Renée come in.

'Hello, my favourite girl,' Bill calls up the stairs. 'You're ravishing, my dear. I almost wish I was the lucky groom.'

'Yes,' adds Renée, 'very pretty, my dear, very, very pretty.'

I can't help smiling as I begin my slow and stately descent.

Stephen, emerging from the back room with Dad, doesn't ruffle my hair as he usually does, but pats me awkwardly on the shoulder instead and says, 'You look so grown up, I hardly recognise our little Lucy.' Even on my wedding day I find I have time to feel slightly annoyed by this. After all, *he's* the little brother.

Dad just murmurs, 'Lovely.' He takes my hand and squeezes it. I can feel him trembling.

The bridal car sweeps to a stop opposite the church door, and the two ushers, Alec and Tim, come over to help Dad get out. Julie opens the front passenger door. I step out, and Julie picks up the long folds of my dress. My stomach lurches and sinks. What if Harry isn't here?

I hear Julie whispering to Stephen, 'Your dad OK?', and Stephen whispering back, 'Just about.'

I take my bouquet – it is made up of pink rosebuds – from Julie. Then hand in hand, father and daughter enter the church just in time to hear the vicar say, 'We will greet the bride with the first hymn, "Lead Us, Heavenly Father, Lead Us".' As the organ plays the opening chords, Dad and I begin to walk down the nave.

The hymn over, Laurence Denton announces, 'We are gathered here this afternoon to solemnise the marriage of Lucy and Harry.' He pauses, then continues, 'But first, I must ask that if anyone knows of any just cause or impediment why this man and this woman may not be joined in holy matrimony, you are to declare it now, or forever hold your peace.'

Silence. I bet Mum wishes there were an impediment. She has done all she can to stop this wedding from happening, but now it's too late. I smile beneath my veil.

Laurence asks, 'Who gives this woman to be married to this man?'

Dad, his hand still trembling, puts my hand into Harry's. Thank you, Dad.

'Please be seated,' resumes the vicar, and everyone sits down as Harry squeezes my hand. Of course he's here. How could I have ever doubted that?

'Repeat after me: I, Henry Paul, take thee, Lucy Eleanor Mary, to be my wedded wife. To have and to hold from this day forward…to love and to cherish, till death do us part…'

'I, Lucy Eleanor Mary, take thee, Henry Paul…'

'With this ring, I thee wed. With my body, I thee worship. With all my worldly goods, I thee endow…'

'Now you can put the ring on Lucy's finger.'

Harry slides the ring up to my knuckle and gives it a gentle, tentative push. If you don't push it harder than that, we'll be here all day. I wonder if I should help. But he might not like that. Then with a bit of a wriggle he manages to slip it over my knuckle and up to the base of my finger.

'You may now kiss the bride.'

Harry bends down and our lips meet.

Then somehow, we are in the vestry – I have no idea how we got here – and I am signing the register: Lucy Ansel. We come out of the vestry to Beethoven's sonorous tune, and as we reach the church door, the bells ring out. A flash catches us unawares, and the click of a camera shutter.

Mum later maintains that the black-and-white newspaper photo is the best of the wedding pictures. 'You had your eyes open, Lucy.'

'Yes, Mum, it was sheer vanity. I didn't want to be wearing my sunglasses although the light was so bright.'

There seem to be so many people to meet. Harry's sister Lily gives me a lucky horseshoe, which she has tied with a loop of silk ribbon that she slips over my arm. I nearly stagger beneath its weight, but I manage a thank-you.

'It's from one of my late husband's ponies.'

'Oh, thank you, Lily,' I say once again, thinking, That's a bit strange!

Harry's brothers Peter and Arnold are here too, with their families.

Across the road in the Free Church Hall, Harry and I stand just inside the door, greeting the guests, while Julie, Jill and Dan collect gifts and cards and pile them on a table next to the cake. People stand about in small groups, chatting and sipping sherry. Dad has begged not to be obliged to give a speech, so we have decided that only Harry will speak.

Harry ends his speech with an admission: 'Life hasn't always been easy, and when I lost my beloved Amy two years ago, I was devastated. In fact, I decided to turn up my toes and join her. But then I met Lucy, and I changed my mind. I know it's difficult for Lucy's family to give up their primary role of cherishing her, but I can assure them that I will do everything I can to make her happy, and to support her in her studies. I'll stop here, so that we can all sample the cake. Otherwise, my wife and I might miss our honeymoon train.'

Then, to my surprise, there seems to be another speaker. 'I promise not to keep you long,' he starts, and I recognise his voice at once. 'Harry agreed that I could say a few words. I first became aware of Lucy when she was only thirteen. She sent me the first Braille letter I ever received, after she had heard me talking about how it felt to go blind. I remember that as if it were yesterday. I was impressed then, and I am even more impressed now. I wish

Lucy and Harry every happiness in this new adventure they are embarking on.'

'Now,' says Mum, 'you should cut the cake together for luck.' And she places our hands together on the knife.

Part Four

1

What can I say about our honeymoon in Shropshire, except that it is blissful? I love everything about it, from the double bed so comfortable I feel like a princess ('A queen,' Harry corrects me; 'after all, you're a married woman now'), to the breakfast porridge onto which I trickle honey from The Old Rectory's own bees, to the ham sandwiches and hard-boiled eggs we're given as packed lunches to eat in the garden or sitting on a bench by the river that rolls along only ten minutes' walk from the hotel.

The week is over all too soon, and then we're back in London. How will Harry feel about leaving his Stockwell flat and moving to Coventry? He has lived in London for thirty-two years, since long before he went blind, and the flat and the whole area must be full of memories of Amy. But he assures me that he is happy to move.

It all happens very suddenly. The upstairs neighbour usually reads us our post, but he is away for a few days, and when he gets back we find a letter from the housing department saying that a flat has become available, but we have to give our answer within the week. We take the coach to Coventry the very next day, and are taken to see the flat by Bert Edwards. It is exactly what we want: a ground-floor flat with a small lawn outside. We say yes at once, and after two days of frantic packing, Jean and Tony drive us to Coventry from London, through a rainstorm that is like a monsoon.

We spend the first night with Bert and his wife Barbara, and in the morning they drop us off at our new flat to await the arrival of the removals van. I'm in the kitchen taking stuff out of a box so that I can make us a pot of tea when I hear a knock at the door.

Harry calls out, 'I'll go,' and I hear the door opening and a woman's voice asking, 'Mr Ansel?'

'Yes.'

'I'm Andrea Dennis, a social worker. I heard you were moving in here today, and thought I'd come and see how you are managing.' I don't hear Harry inviting her to come in, but now she seems to be in the living room. 'No furniture yet?' she asks.

'We're expecting the van at around two,' says Harry.

I walk in. 'Who is it, darling?'

'I'm a social worker, Andrea Dennis.'

I politely offer her a cup of tea, although I can't imagine what she's doing here.

'There's only one chair at present,' says Harry, 'and that's Lucy's.'

Andrea Dennis takes the mug of tea I offer, and asks rudely, 'What's your cooker: gas or electric?'

'Electric,' I say.

'Got an electrician to install it?'

'Yes,' says Harry. 'Me.'

'Oh no, that's not safe: a blind man wiring up an electric cooker.' She moves towards the door. 'Not safe at all. I'll go and fetch one.'

We wonder who alerted social services. I really hope they're not going to keep hanging around, trying to interfere.

Just then we hear a van pulling up outside, and then there comes a knock on the door. It's the furniture van: they bring in the cooker first, and Harry gets to work on it while they unload everything else.

The next knock brings Uncle Bill and Aunt Renée. Harry and Renée hang the curtains, and Bill reads out the labels on the boxes while I unpack and put things away. We have just about finished when there's another knock at the door.

'That'll be the social worker,' says Harry, and he opens the door to find Andrea Dennis and an electrician. 'The cooker's already wired in,' he tells her.

'But I must get it checked.'

Harry sighs. 'Be my guest.' And he leads the way to the kitchen.

'Well,' says the electrician ten minutes later, 'it's done perfectly. I couldn't do a better job myself. How on earth did you manage it with no sight?'

'We have our methods,' says Harry, as I smother a laugh.

2

I've missed the first few days of term, and now I have to learn the route to and from the college. I learn to go past our flat on the way home and down to the kerb on Torrington Avenue, then turn around and count back ten paces, which brings me to a spot directly opposite our garden path. Monty Davison, Wake College's mobility officer, comes over and teaches Harry the way to and from the shops, including, importantly, the fish and chip shop.

'So, you're back,' says Mr Longbourne when he sees me at my desk in his English class. 'We've been reading Aldous Huxley's *Brave New World*, do you know it?'

'I read it some years ago, but I don't remember much detail, just some of the sayings: "The tot is in the pot", "The more stitches, the less riches." Oh, and the infamous "soma holidays".'

I have to reread it, and Mr Longbourne wants me to read up a bit on the philosophy of utilitarianism so as to broaden my understanding of it. He recommends Bertrand Russell's take on it in *A History of Western Philosophy*. I feel as if I have some considerable catching up to do.

I find it quite tiring being back at college and having to go to and fro rather than living there in the hostel, but oh, the joy of coming home each evening to a warm flat and Harry's warm arms! The move appears to have released Harry's inner carpenter: he tells me he loves the way that carpentry involves the hands and brain working together. In no time at all he has installed built-in wardrobes and folding doors throughout the flat.

In my first piano lesson I play the last piece I learned.

'Not bad, considering you haven't been able to play since you broke up for the summer,' says Shirley Dyson.

I tell her that my piano is coming over from Bentham Close this very day.

'That'll be good. I think you should carry on learning your grade six pieces.'

'Are you sure I'll be ready to take grade six next spring?'

'I don't see why not. You might have trouble with some of the arpeggios, but you should be able to manage most of them well enough. Anyway, that's enough for today. Are you going home now?'

'Yes.'

'Want a lift?'

'Please – then you can come in and meet Harry.'

That Saturday we are expecting our first visit from Mum; she is being driven over by Uncle Bill. When they ring the new doorbell – installed by Harry – Harry lets them in and brings them into the sitting room while I get tea ready in the kitchen.

'You've got the settee and the table in the wrong places,' I hear Mum say. 'The settee should be under the window and the table in the middle of the room.'

In the kitchen, I am cringing. Here we go. I put together the tea tray and carry it through.

'I'll take that,' says Mum, grabbing it from me and putting it on the table, then walking into the kitchen to fetch the teapot. 'I'm Mum,' she says as she pours the tea.

Too right you are. But whose flat is this? Harry squeezes my hand.

'I like the folding door,' says Mum. 'I could do with one of those in my kitchen.'

'I'll get you one and fix it next time we're over,' Harry says.

'You? But you can't do things like that.' Mum speaks as if this is a statement of fact.

'Well,' says Bill, 'Harry did that one and the one for the box room. He's also dismantled a wardrobe and used the wood to make a built-in wardrobe with a cupboard above it.'

'I'll show you round when you've finished your tea,' says Harry.

Mum is silent for a moment. She must be looking out of the window, because then she says, 'There's a nice load of washing on a line out there. It's blowing well in the breeze.'

'Lucy did that in our new washing machine,' says Harry. 'I put the line up yesterday while she was at college.'

3

I am surprised at how quickly Harry and I slip into a comfortable routine. We share our domestic tasks according to ability and inclination. I draw up the shopping lists and I'm in charge of the cooking. After our evening meal, I wash up while Harry dries and puts the dishes away; then I relax in my armchair while he makes a pot of tea, which we drink while listening to *The Archers*. On Tuesday and Thursday evenings a reader from Bert Edwards's service comes to help me with my college work. On Mondays Harry has a reader to help him deal with general post and bills, and I have a late evening class at college. One rainy Monday evening Tim, who is Harry's reader that day, insists on picking me up from college, and that too becomes routine with all the readers, so that I'm always picked up on a Monday and dropped off at the flat. Is everything going too swimmingly? Sometimes I hear a little whisper in the corner of my mind: when is it going to go wrong? When will the arguments begin?

'What a load of rubbish,' says Harry one evening as he switches off *The Hitchhiker's Guide to the Galaxy*.

'It's not rubbish! In fact, I think it's very clever.'

Harry laughs and laughs. 'At last. I wondered when you were going to stop agreeing with everything I say and playing the perfect wife. A perfect wife like that is not the Lucy I know and love.'

*

'Your mother won't be able to move the table if we lay out all the crockery on it beforehand,' says Harry. 'And if we put Jill and Dan on the sofa, she won't be able to move that, either.'

It is another Saturday afternoon, and we are awaiting the arrival of Mum and Dad, Stephen and Rosemary (not the kids this first time), and Jill and Dan, for our first ceremonial tea party to show that we are fully moved in. Harry is trying to make me laugh, I know, because he knows how anxious I'm feeling. Unusually for me, my nervousness has manifested in my baking: one burned sponge cake has had to be binned, and a second one, a coffee sponge, has mysteriously refused to rise. I am just about to bin that one too when Harry, attracted by the smell, comes into the kitchen and demands to try it.

'Mmm, it's delicious,' he says. 'A little bit crunchy, but let's cut it up, and you can tell them it's home-made coffee biscuits.'

'OK,' I say, but I send him out for a shop-bought Victoria sponge, just in case.

When the doorbell rings I open the door and welcome everyone in. I show them where the hooks are to hang their coats, and then I take Dad's hand and lead the way to the sitting room. 'Here, Dad, you can sit at this end of the table next to me. Mum can sit opposite, next to Harry. Rosemary and Jill here, and, Dan and Stephen, you'll have to sit on the sofa. The tea's made.'

'I'll fetch it through,' says Mum immediately.

'No,' says Harry, 'you're our guest today: I'll bring the teapot in. But if you like, you can pour.'

Well done, Harry. Mum is appeased.

Harry goes out and comes back with two plates of sandwiches. 'There's salmon and cucumber, or egg and tomato,' he says, putting the plates down in the middle of the table.

'I love your decor,' says Jill. 'It's fresh and very modern.'

'But surely,' says Mum, 'there ought to be a patterned wallpaper in a living room?'

'I think the trend for plain painted walls is great,' says Rosemary. 'There's enough of a pattern in the curtains.'

I smile to myself. It's almost as if Jill and Rosemary are reading from a script. It's perfect! Soon we are all eating peaches and cream, which go down well with everyone.

Dan gets up from the sofa and looks out of the window. 'I thought you said the grass was a mess. It looks neat enough to me.'

'Well,' says Harry, 'Bert's lawnmower was able to do a decent cut once I removed some of the jungle by hand.'

I slip off to the kitchen and come back with a plate in each hand. 'Cake or biscuits for anyone?' I offer. 'The sponge isn't home-made, I'm afraid, but the coffee biscuits are.'

'I'll refill the teapot,' says Mum.

'That's my job,' says Harry.

'These biscuits are scrumptious,' says Dad. 'Please may I have another?'

Both Jill and Rosemary ask me for the recipe. I am not quite sure that I should admit that they started off as a cake. Perhaps I'll pretend they were meant to be biscuits all along.

4

September 1975, I am almost thirty-one, and it's the beginning of my final year at Wake College. I'm taking A levels in English and history, grade six piano, and (now that Mr Brandon has taught himself Braille over the summer) O level maths. I need the maths if I want to go to university. I'll still have to teach him how to use a Taylor frame, but I know that he's a fast learner. If I – ever! – get to university, I'd like to study philosophy; I blame Mr Longbourne and Bertrand Russell for that. And maybe – who knows? – those first walks I took on my own, before I ever met Harry, along roads and avenues called Pascal, Hume and Kant. I wonder who decided to name those little suburban streets after a bunch of philosophers?

In the New Year, Harry's really pleased to hear that the Guide Dogs for the Blind Association think they have found him a suitable dog: he is to go for training in the early summer. At the same time Mr Lockhead arranges for me to go and have a talk with Dr Stone, the head of philosophy at the University of Warwick. We get on well. He explains that as a mature student I could be offered an unconditional place, but they would want to see good grades in my A levels, and a minimum C in O level maths. Otherwise, he says, I'll struggle with mathematical logic, which is a requirement in the first year of philosophy, and has to be passed in order to stay on the course. I do not get on so well with the man in charge of the university's medical service. He doesn't actually say it outright, but I suspect that he believes that people with disabilities like mine should be kept out of the public eye, and should on no account attempt a university education.

I feel really distressed, not least because I assume that he has the power to let me in or keep me out. I mean, he's a doctor, and in my experience doctors are very powerful men. I resign myself to being turned down. It was a stupid dream in the first place, I tell myself. How could someone like me ever hope to go to university? What an idiot I've been. But the next week the phone rings, and it's Dr Stone himself, with an offer of a place on the philosophy degree course, subject to acceptable grades. There are two conditions, he tells me, that the head of the medical service has insisted on: I am not to live on campus, and I am not to sign up with the university's medical service. Dr Stone sounds embarrassed as he states these conditions. He says he's really sorry. I can't help laughing. 'I never want to see that man again,' I tell Dr Stone. 'I found him extremely insulting. As for living on campus, I'm happy here in my flat with my husband. Why on earth should I want to live on campus?'

'So you agree to the conditions?'

'Absolutely.'

5

'Harry, what are you doing?'

'Putting your white coat on you.' He places my long cane in my hand, hustles me out of the front door, and quickly shuts it. Then he opens the letter flap and calls through it, 'You're not coming back in here until you've got a new coat.'

I am stunned and bewildered. What? I stand motionless. There's something in my right-hand pocket. I put my hand in there and find a roll of banknotes. But no door key. I hammer on the door. 'Let me in, let me in!'

The letter flap opens once again. 'No, not without a new coat. You're not a child and I'm not buying it for you. I'm your husband, not your mother. Go on, I know you can do it.'

'Sod you,' I scream. But what can I do? I stamp up and down for a bit, then I set off for the bus stop. How dare he, how dare he shut me out like that?

Tu-ta, tu-ta, tu-ta. Is that an engine ticking over? A lorry or a—

'Are you catching this bus?' calls the conductor.

After clambering on board, I slide into the first seat, fearful but still shaking with anger.

'Where to, miss?'

I snap, 'It's Mrs, actually.' Then I soften my voice and hold out my pass. 'Corporation Street, please.'

When I get off, fear clutches at my bowels. There's a raging torrent of traffic here, and all the shops are on the other side. I'll never get across alone. I take a few steps and come to a halt.

'Want to cross?' quavers an old woman.

'Ye… Yes, please.'

Taking my hand in trembling, gnarled fingers, the woman says, 'We can cross now.'

Who's helping who? I wonder briefly.

'Where're you going?' she asks when we reach the far pavement.

Oh dear, I don't know who sells coats. 'Do you know the way to Marks & Spencer?' I ask.

Turning to her left, the woman raises the tip of my cane and points it. 'Go down there, and turn right just before that green building.'

I hear her footsteps retreating. What green building? Does she think my white stick's a fashion statement, or what? I set off in the direction indicated but, after a while, I falter to a stop again.

A man asks in a musical baritone, 'What are you looking for?'

'M&S.'

'Turn right at the end of this building, and you're nearly there.'

Reaching the corner, I am buffeted by a gust of wind and a flurry of dead leaves. It feels as though it's going to rain. I shiver. That's all I need. Turning the corner, I walk on a short way, and again I hover, forlorn.

'Ooh, look, Mummy: a faerwee with a wand,' pipes up a small child.

'No, Melissa,' laughs a young woman. 'That's not a wand. It's a blind lady's stick.' Then she asks if she can help.

Again I ask for Marks & Spencer, and she tells me it's three doors down on the right. I thank her and move to the building line.

'Bye-bye, faerwee,' calls the little girl after me.

I count three doors and my hearing aid picks up a hum. I reach out and push open a door, and creep inside. I'll look really stupid if they don't sell coats, but here goes.

'Can I help, madam?'

Keeping my voice low, I ask, 'Do you sell winter coats?'

'Certainly, madam. One moment, and I'll get an assistant.'

In a few moments my hand is taken in a warm, plump hold, and a matronly woman says, 'We'll go up in the lift.' Then, stepping out, she says, 'Ladies' coats are this way. What kind of coat would you like, dearie?'

'What kind of coats have you got?'

'Ah, I'll go and see.' And her footsteps fade away.

'Can I help?' This is a younger woman.

'It's all right, Mavis. I'm seeing to this lady. I've got two coats for you to try. One's camel hair with a hood, or there's this red coat.'

I suppose I should buy the camel hair. It's probably more serviceable and hard-wearing, but…

'The red one would suit you, dearie, with your dark hair.'

I smile. 'OK. Let's try them both on.'

'The camel hair is nice, and it makes you look smart,' comments the assistant, 'but the red really does look absolutely smashing on you.'

'How much is the red one?'

'Twenty-five pounds.'

I pull the roll of fivers from my pocket, and count one, two, three, four, five. The exact amount. A thrill of pleasure sets my pulse dancing. I take a deep breath and declare, 'I'll have the red one, please.'

'Will you wear it, dearie, or take it in a bag?'

'I'll wear it.' I don't ever want to wear this horrid white coat again.

Slowly, hesitantly, I retrace my steps to the bus stop, but I can't stop myself grinning like the Cheshire cat. When I get home I rap briskly on the door.

The letter flap opens. 'Got a coat?'

Now I bang on the door and yell, 'Let me in, or else.'

The door opens and I throw myself into Harry's arms.

'I did it, I did it,' I murmur into his neck as his arms tighten around me.

'I knew, I *knew* you could do it.'

I kiss him, and a warm wave of triumph sweeps through me.

And then the exams start. And with them, a dose of hay fever such as I have never experienced before. Dr Bramley offers me an antihistamine, but when he tells me it might cause drowsiness and irritability, I decide not to take it. I daren't. I need all my faculties for these exams.

Twenty-three hours over two weeks, and because one of the maths papers clashes with an English paper (there can't be many people doing A levels at the same time as O levels), I have to spend one night in isolation at the college so as to take the English paper the following day, after everyone else has done it.

I'll be so glad when they're all over. There's something funny going on in Bentham Close, but I daren't ask what. I've got to stay focused on these exams. So much depends on them. Well, everything, really.

*

Somehow, with the aid of countless boxes of tissues, I get through my exams. I am feeling bone-tired. It's the day of my final exam: a history paper. My nose is still streaming, and my eyes are hot and itchy. I have written my answer to the first question when the typewriter suddenly jams. I check the hammers, but they're not stuck; I try to force the carriage back, but it refuses to budge. I call the invigilator from the adjoining room: there's a problem with the ribbon. A phone call to the exam board, they agree that my clock can be stopped, someone is dispatched to get a new ribbon, and after what seems like an eternity I can get going again.

I get home very late that evening.

'You must be completely done in,' says Harry, hugging me as I come through the front door.

'Yes, I am. But they're all over now. Hooray! Nothing I can do now except wait for the results.' I flop onto the sofa. 'Now, please tell me what's going on at home.'

Harry sits down beside me and puts his arms around me. 'I'm afraid your dad's in hospital. He had another coronary on Tuesday. He's better than he was, but he's still in intensive care.'

I rest my head on Harry's shoulder. 'I knew something was up, but I had to block it out. Does that seem heartless?'

'No, darling. He'll understand. You've worked so hard, and he wouldn't want to jeopardise your chances of getting into university.'

We kiss for a long time. Then I say, 'I knew you'd understand, but I must go over there today.'

'Don't worry,' says my Harry. 'Bert said to ring as soon as you were ready, and he'll drive us over there now.'

*

As I walk into the ward, I hear the *bleep, bleep* of the heart monitors and my pulse begins to race in response. I take Dad's hand in mine. 'Dad, I'm here now.'

I feel a feeble pressure: good, at least he knows I'm here.

Mum hugs me. 'I've been so worried.'

I return her embrace. 'I know, Mum. I'm sorry. But thank you for letting me do the exams.'

6

The maths O level result comes first: I get a B. The A level results come a week later: an A in English but, disappointingly, only an E in history. I think my university chances must be scuppered, but Mr Lockhead is sure it'll be all right, and tells me to ring Dr Stone at Warwick for confirmation. Dr Stone reassures me: the offer of a place was unconditional apart from the maths, but anyway, he says, even with the points system I'd be in: A and E count for more than B and D, for example. With my B in O level maths, there is, therefore, no problem.

It is a happy summer. Slowly but steadily, Dad recovers from his heart attack, and once a week we go over to Milton and play dominoes or Monopoly with him. We also take a wonderful week's holiday in a farmhouse in Devon.

When we get back I invite Mum and Dad, along with Bill and Renée, over for a meal to celebrate my university place. To my surprise, Dad boldly requests a curry. I'm really happy to get the opportunity to cook the chicken curry that I made under Miss Winter's supervision at Wake College, and which was eaten with such relish by Mohammed, Dave and Jo; so I don't mind having to cook a separate dish – a cottage pie – for the less adventurous Mum and Renée. Bill follows Dad's lead and opts for the curry.

Over dinner Harry tells everyone that after a few delays he has, at last, got a dog lined up for him by the Guide Dogs

Association, and that the two of them will start training at the Leamington centre on 6 October.

He's barely finished talking about it when Mum says, 'You'll have to come and stay with us, Lucy, while Harry's in Leamington.'

'I can't do that, Mum. I'm starting at the university on the same day.'

'But you can't stay here by yourself.'

'She'll be fine,' says Harry. 'She'll eat at the university each day, then most evenings she'll have a reader over.'

'But—'

'No, Mary,' says Dad. 'Lucy's a grown woman, and a married one. She can't keep running home all the time.'

7

6 October 1976. Today both of us are new bugs: me at the university, and Harry at the guide dog training centre. I won't deny that I'm a bit worried about living on my own in the flat for a whole month, but, as we say our goodbyes, I am more worried about what faces me at the university.

I cling to Harry in the hallway. 'I'm going to miss you. A month's a long time to be apart.'

An arrangement has been made whereby I'll get picked up each morning at 8.45 by the minibus that takes a group of cleaners to the university. As I'm clinging to Harry in the hallway we hear the bus's *beep*, *beep* outside.

'Here she comes,' chorus the women as I come out of the front door, and as I climb aboard I'm greeted with 'Hello, dear' and 'Hello, my lovely.'

I smile at the warmth of this welcome, but my stomach is churning. It'll be all right, I tell myself, it'll be all right.

The minibus drops me just outside the arts and social science building, and I find my way to the philosophy common room, where all of us first-years have been instructed to gather. I am relieved to hear the calm voice of Dr Stone, who explains the induction routine, talks about timetables, and introduces me to the group, asking them all to look out for me until I find my way around. Then we are sent off for a tour of the department, and to the library to register. Everyone gets up to go, and someone taps me lightly on the shoulder.

'Hello,' says a young woman. 'My name's Katy Bratton – would you like me to guide you?'

'Yes, please.'

'How do you like to be guided?'

'Slip your hand under my right arm. I'm too short to do the usual elbow hold.'

We set off, and I explain to Katy that I don't live on campus, and that I'm married and live in a flat in Coventry with my husband. Katy is good at guiding. Most people manage to bump me into doorways. She tells me that her father is blind, so she's had lots of practice.

The university chaplaincy has organised a rota of people to drive me home in the evenings at six o'clock. That first evening alone at home is long and lonely, especially after a phone call with Harry during which we swap our first-day experiences. Harry tells me about Tessa, his black Labrador, who, he says, seems very gentle and intelligent.

After I've spoken to Harry I start to get things ready for the morning: the Brailled timetable, the small recorder, the microphone. Then I tidy away my books. Suddenly I think, What am I doing? I'm just putting off going to bed – an empty bed in an empty flat – but I can't stay up for a month. I've got to sleep sometime. Stop being silly, Lucy, I say to myself, and I get undressed and go to bed.

When I wake up the next morning, I think, What was that all about, then? Nothing happened: the flat didn't go up in flames, and nobody broke in to murder me in my bed. I get dressed and have breakfast, and I'm waiting outside with all my things when the minibus pulls up.

The days fall into a pattern of lectures and study. Because I don't have a room on campus, I've been given a key to one of the study carrels in the library. It's quite small and there isn't room enough to keep all of my Braille books there, so each day I have to lug in whichever volumes I need. Katy is a great support, and introduces me to others in our year. The Roman Catholic chaplain, Father Hollywell, who organised the evening lift rota, searches me out and we have a chat about this and that. He seems like a nice person.

It's my birthday on Saturday. I'm going to be thirty-two. Tim rings the evening before, and suggests he pick me up from campus and drive me over to Leamington to visit Harry at the training centre. Usually visitors aren't allowed for the first fortnight, but it seems that Harry's trainer is keen for me to meet up with Tessa the Labrador, as she is going to be a part of my life as well as Harry's. Or perhaps that is a little bit of an excuse; I gather Harry has been talking about how much he is missing his wife.

When Tim and I arrive, we are met in the car park by Harry's trainer, a man called Darren Carter, who explains that he's a bit worried because of Tessa's liking to stand up and lick people's faces. I agree that such a move could easily knock me flat on my back. We go up together to Harry's room, and after knocking, Darren goes in first, then calls to me to come in. I walk in and stand still, and then I feel a soft, wet pressure on the back of one of my hands, followed after a short pause by a creak.

'Well, if I hadn't seen that happen I wouldn't have believed it,' says Darren.

'What happened?' asks Harry.

'Tessa walked over to your wife, licked her hand, then went back to her bed. I think you should give Tessa a reward and some praise for that. It seems you're going to be all right, so I'll leave you for half an hour. Only half an hour though, then Mrs Ansel must leave.'

The door shuts, and Harry has his arms around me. 'Happy birthday, darling, happy birthday. Come and sit next to me on the bed.'

'Oh, Harry!' I kiss him hard. 'I've really, really missed you.'

'Me too you,' he says, showering my face with kisses. 'Now, let me introduce you properly. Tessa, come here.'

The dog bed creaks and the next minute Tessa is licking my hand again, and then, when we sit down, she lays her head on my lap. Suddenly I'm back with Miss Armstrong, learning Braille for the very first time with Sheba's head in my lap. I haven't thought about this before, but I realise now that I am very pleased that another dog is coming into my life.

8

Once Harry is home with Tessa the weeks fly by. I look forward every morning to the day ahead, to the lectures and seminars and chats with my fellow students, and every afternoon I look forward to the evening at home: to cooking dinner and eating it with Harry, to reading with Tim or one of the other readers, and to sitting on the sofa with Harry's arm around me, listening to a concert on the radio or to one of our LPs.

Exams come, and exams go. Soon I have completed my first year of studying philosophy at the University of Warwick.

During the summer vacation, the department of philosophy moves into one of the university's brand-new buildings. The week before term starts, I get a call from Dr Stone, suggesting I come in before the start of term so that he can show me around the new building. I have a good rapport with Dr Stone.

He shows me the side entrance to the new building, and directs me up the two flights of stairs that lead to the department. We go to his new office, and over a cup of tea he tells me that as the next-door office is currently empty, they have made it over for me to use as a study.

'There are plenty of shelves big enough to take Braille volumes, so you won't need to carry so much to and from home.'

I am really touched by Dr Stone's consideration and kindness. I almost cry, but manage to stop myself. 'Thank you,' I say. 'That'll be a real help. I'm not sure how I manage to carry so much. The other day Harry weighed my Karrimor, and we were both shocked when the scales said thirty-two pounds.'

Dr Stone hands me a key, which I slip into my pocket. A key to my very own study!

There is one problem with the new building: a bridge that links two sides of the upper storeys.

'I want to show you the bridge while it's quiet,' Dr Stone tells me, 'because I'm a bit worried that it's dangerous. There's a large gap between the handrail and the floor. The powers that be say it's all right as children aren't allowed in the building, but they seem to have overlooked short people and the blind. I could say "Avoid it altogether", but it's the only way to reach the public telephones and the drinks machines. Besides which, by crossing it you can get almost all the way to the chaplaincy without going outside. Shall we go and try it?'

As we walk down the corridor he tells me that he has made an official complaint on behalf of the department. He tells me to follow the right-hand wall until I come to a glass door, which he holds open for me. Now we're in the politics department, and the next glass door, he tells me, opens onto the bridge. Once we're through that one, he takes my left arm and taps my cane on the edge of the bridge.

'The handrail is just below your shoulder height,' he says.

I see exactly what he means about the danger. I'll have to be very, very careful. I determine to ring the mobility officer about it as soon as I get home.

Towards the end of the autumn term, two distressing events occur. The first takes place in Dr Holden's seminar on political philosophy.

At the end of the seminar, a boy called Roger says to Dr Holden, in a whining tone of voice, 'You don't like me. You always give Lucy higher marks than me, and she's not even a Marxist.'

'Grow up, Roger,' says Dr Holden angrily.

'But you do.'

'Well, at least Lucy is prepared to argue her corner using philosophical ideas. You're behaving like a spoiled brat.'

'You can't call me a brat.'

'I didn't. I said you were behaving like one.'

Roger continues to bluster, throwing around phrases like 'special treatment' and 'favouritism'. I feel increasingly uncomfortable, and eventually get up and leave the seminar room, my face burning.

A few days after that unpleasantness, I am unlocking my study door when a student called Marianna, whom I have always found friendly, comes up to me and asks if she can come in and have a look at my study.

'Of course.'

She walks over to the window, where she stands in silence for a minute, and then suddenly bursts out with 'It's not fair. Why should you have a room of your own? A room with a lovely view?' She rushes past me and out, and slams the door behind her.

I stagger to my chair. I am shaking all over. I had no idea that my fellow students were so angry and hostile towards me. And what good does Marianna think a lovely view is to me? I try to turn the thought into a joke, but it doesn't work.

When there's a knock at the door a bit later, and I call out, 'Come in,' I can hear the tremble in my voice.

Katy comes in, bearing two cups of tea, and I tell her about Marianna's outburst, and what Roger said the other day.

Roger, says Katy, is well known for his resentment of the students who do better than he does. 'The fact is, he's really lazy. But he thinks he's really clever.'

'And Marianna?'

'I don't know,' says Katy. 'I think they've both got problems of their own, and they're quick to blame other people. Though why they should pick on you, I don't know…'

'It's because I'm different,' I say.

Early in the New Year, snow falls, and turns the campus white for nearly a fortnight. I hate snow; it's like fog under your feet. I have to pick my way across campus with the utmost care, poking my stick into the snow, looking for kerbs and other obstacles. Thank goodness for shoe chains. As soon as I'm inside the philosophy building, I bend over to remove the chains.

'Aha – cheating, I see,' says Dr Holden, coming in behind me one day. 'I've been watching you for days, wondering why you're the only person on campus who hasn't yet fallen over. Now I know!'

I laugh. I like Dr Holden.

'By the way, Monica tells me you haven't visited the careers department yet.'

'There's no point,' I say. 'An adviser at the RNIB says I'm unemployable.'

'What rot. You've got one of the best attendance records on campus. You even turn up in all this snow. You know, plenty of able-bodied students are ringing in saying they can't make it, but not you. I think you really should go and have a talk with someone in careers. I believe you're going to go far.'

*

The snow has been gone for a week or so when I get home one evening and am met at the door by Harry, who tells me not to worry (I immediately feel hugely anxious), but he had a fall earlier, and a policeman will be coming round soon as a result. What? I am beside myself with worry, but Harry makes me sit down, gets me a cup of tea, and then tells me what happened. The whole thing was really his fault, he says, because he ignored Tessa's warning signs. They were walking along with some shopping when suddenly she sat down and refused to budge.

'I thought she was playing up,' says Harry sadly.

'But she doesn't usually play up, does she?'

'No – I don't know what I was thinking. But I forced her on, and we both fell into a trench, which had gravel in the bottom.'

'Oh, Harry!' I put my arms around him. 'Poor you, and poor Tessa.'

'She's OK,' says Harry. He tells me how she scrambled out of the trench and barked for help, and then accompanied him to A&E, where they cleaned the gravel out of his face and hands.

'Oh, my love!' I feel so upset I start to cry.

Again Harry says, 'It was my own fault, and I'm not badly hurt – just grazed and a bit stiff.'

Just then, the doorbell goes. A young constable comes in and tells us that the hole that Harry fell into should have been barriered off. A barrier has now been erected, with warning lights at either end. 'It wasn't your fault, sir,' says the constable.

Later, when we're sitting side by side on the sofa with our arms around each other and listening to Schubert on the record player, Harry says, 'It *was* my fault, you know. I should have trusted Tessa.'

Two weeks pass and Harry is still stiff and aching after his fall. He goes to the GP, who tells him that he probably pulled some muscles when he fell. He advises Harry to take aspirin and keep exercising. Another few weeks pass and Harry is still in pain. The GP sends him for an X-ray, but it reveals nothing untoward. Spring turns to summer. Harry gets out the lawnmower and extends his daily walks with Tessa, but I know that he is still in pain, and that the aspirin doesn't touch it.

Meanwhile, I have taken Dr Holden's advice and been to see Monica in the university's careers department. I've told her that I would be interested in teaching or the law. I am aware that both of these fields require further qualifications: a teacher training course for the former; a law conversion course for the latter. However, Monica is very encouraging and offers to make enquiries on my behalf. She starts with the teacher training course at the polytechnic. The response is swift and brutal: they won't even consider interviewing me. That setback only seems to make Monica more determined, and in her research on my behalf she discovers the existence of an Association of Blind Lawyers. I write to them at their London address, and ask if there is someone I could go to talk to about a career as a lawyer.

A couple of weeks later, I receive a letter inviting me to meet a Miss Mullen at the association's offices in Lincoln's Inn. The evening before I go to London, I urge Harry to go back to the GP and ask for a referral.

'He hasn't done anything since he sent you for that X-ray four months ago,' I say as I stroke his arm. It's very hard to ask for things, but sometimes you just have to keep on doing it.

Deborah Mullen, it turns out, is a straight-talking woman. 'The first thing I must say,' she begins, 'is never write another letter like the one you sent me. Of course, we have to be honest about our handicaps, but we need to be careful how we present ourselves.'

'What did I do wrong?'

'Setting it out in such a blunt way in the first sentence: "I am a multiply handicapped woman…"'

'OK, what should I have done?' I ask.

'A good letter begins with positive things, like "I am a mature student in the second year of a philosophy degree, and considering law as a career." You should also finish on an up note: something along the lines of why you are interested in the law. Then when you describe your handicaps it is important to show how you overcome any problems. For instance: "Although I cannot drive, I am an independent user of public transport. My written and verbal communication skills are good, and I have a variety of ways of dealing with written work, including by using readers."'

'I see,' I say. And I do.

'The most important thing to remember is that if you describe your handicaps at the beginning of a letter, most people won't read any further.' She pauses. 'On the other hand,' and I hear the smile in her voice, 'if that is the last thing you say, it is the only part of your letter they will remember, and it will go straight in the wastepaper basket.'

Goodness me. I hadn't thought about it like that. How very tricky!

Deborah goes on to talk in detail, both in practical and in psychological terms, about what is required of a lawyer who is blind. Her overall message is that a blind lawyer has to be twice as good as a sighted one, but that a career in law is not impossible.

9

It is Len the chiropodist who raises the alarm inside my head, or is it just that he confirms what I know, deep down, to be the case? Months have gone by with no let-up in the pain Harry is experiencing. After considerable perseverance he now has an appointment with a rheumatologist.

Len hasn't seen us since before Christmas. Now, in our sitting room, he gets up from the floor. 'Well,' he says, 'you now both have tidy feet again. Harry's nails were like Dracula's. I'll see you both again on…bother, I've left my diary in the car. Lucy, can you come out? I'm in a bit of a rush.'

This is unlike Len, but I follow him out as he suggests.

As soon as the front door is closed behind us, he drops his voice and says, 'I don't want to alarm you, but Harry looks dreadful.'

'He's got an appointment at the hospital next month.'

'I don't think he should wait that long. Could you not get him to be seen sooner?'

But what can I do? Matters are made much worse when the university's Anglican chaplain, Donald Franks, starts to interfere. He takes it upon himself to make enquiries at the surgery, and perhaps because he is a chaplain, or perhaps because he is a smooth talker, he finds out what the GP really thinks is going on, and he relays it to me. Harry, as the GP understands it and vouchsafes to the chaplain, is bored and fretful with me being out at the university all day. He is lonely and frustrated, and is imagining his pains as a distraction.

'In other words,' Donald Franks says to me when I am next in the chaplaincy, 'Harry is malingering and it's being made worse for him by your increasing distress. Lucy, you really must stop working yourself up like this. If you're not careful you'll end up in a mental hospital.'

My blood runs cold. A mental hospital! I am only too aware of how easily people like me can be 'put away'. 'I am not hysterical,' I say quietly, and as calmly as I possibly can. 'I am just worried.'

'I know you don't think Harry eats enough,' says the chaplain casually, 'but people don't when they're older. It's natural and nothing to fret over.'

What on earth does he know about it? I stand up. 'My driver will be waiting for me,' I say, and I leave the room. I feel really shaken. I'll have to stop talking to people about Harry. We'll just have to deal with this on our own. Thank God he's got that hospital appointment next week.

The appointment is on the Friday afternoon. It is inconclusive. They seem to be unable to read the X-ray that's been taken. They ask Harry if he suffers from constipation, and when he says that he does, they give him something to take and say they'll do another X-ray on Monday.

On Monday morning, I wake to an empty space beside me. Where's Harry? There's a funny smell. I slide out of bed and head for the bathroom, where the smell turns into a terrible stink.

'Darling, how long have you...?'

'It feels like hours,' he groans from between chattering teeth.

The doorbell rings. 'Ambulance for Mr Ansel?'

'He's in the bathroom in a bad way. I don't know what to do…'

'All right, Mrs, I'll see. Hold on, laddie. We'll soon get you to the hospital.'

'But I can't stop it…'

'We'll put something in your pants, and get you on a stretcher. You'll feel better lying down.'

I reach into the airing cupboard and grab a pile of hand towels. 'Would these help?'

'Just the ticket, Mrs. I'll call my mate.'

'Shall I come with you in the ambulance, darling?' I ask Harry.

'No, love, you go off to university as usual.'

'If you're sure?'

'Absolutely.'

Dr Fleming has just begun her lecture when I slide into a seat at the back of the hall. She pauses and waits while I switch on my tape recorder. 'To repeat…' she says.

At the end of the lecture she stops on her way out, just as I'm stowing away my recorder.

'Is there something wrong, Lucy? It looked to me as if you were wiping away the odd tear.'

I tell her that Harry has gone into hospital, but I can't tell her the details. My voice is cracking.

'Come along to my room and tell me about it over coffee.'

'I wanted to go with him, but he's so worried about all of this interfering with my degree, especially now, with exams coming up and everything.'

Dr Fleming listens wonderfully. She asks Sarah, the department secretary, to ring the hospital and ask them to ring the department as soon as there is news of Harry.

They keep Harry in hospital for ten days, taking a series of X-rays, each one preceded by a violent enema. I visit every evening during the permitted hour and a half, and Harry always clings on to my hands.

'They think my constipation is to do with my diet,' he tells me. 'The consultant says I should eat All-Bran every morning, and that should do the trick.'

I feel completely helpless. Surely that can't be the problem, but what do I know? Well, I do know quite a lot about hospitals, and how they can sap your dignity and your sense of self.

Harry is brought home by ambulance. I can hear the tiredness in his voice as the ambulance driver brings him in.

'Welcome home, darling.' I try to sound bright and cheerful. 'I was beginning to think they'd lost the way.'

'It's good to be home. The journey in the ambulance was hairy. It felt as if we were bumping along a stony track, and my back really aches.'

'You're home now. Come and sit on the sofa and I'll make you a cup of tea. What would you like for dinner?'

'I'm not very hungry.'

My heart sinks. 'Surely you can manage some fish and chips?'

'OK, I'll try.'

But he doesn't eat much of the fish, and hardly any of the chips, either. When I point this out, he says snappishly, 'I told you I wasn't hungry. I can't eat, or think of anything else except

270

the pain when it's this bad. They sent me home without any painkillers, too.'

I scrape the food into the bin, and do the washing-up as tears run silently down my cheeks. 'I'm sorry, darling, but we haven't got any painkillers here. I'll go and get some first thing in the morning.' I drift towards the bathroom door.

'It's no good going to the bathroom to cry. That won't take my pain away,' Harry says sharply. And then he shouts, 'You don't know what it's like. It's unbearable.'

'And what do you expect me to do?' I shout back at him. Then I cross the room, sit on the sofa, and take one of his hands in both of mine. 'Why are we shouting at each other? We're on the same side, aren't we?'

We are both crying now, arms around each other, clinging together.

10

April drags by. Harry's pain gets worse. I ring the surgery and ask the doctor to call, but I am fobbed off time and again. I don't know what to do. During the day I try to concentrate on my lectures; on reading and revision. Final exams are looming.

One evening at the end of the month Father Hollywell drives me home, and when he asks me how I am, I just burst into tears. I tell him how worried I am about Harry; about how the GP seems to think that Harry is malingering, and that I'm being hysterical. I tell him that Harry is now so weak that he can't even get in and out of the bath, and that the pain is worse than ever. The GP has agreed, reluctantly, to send a nurse round once a week to help him have a bath; and I've been told that he must just carry on with aspirin for the pain.

Two days later Father Hollywell comes and knocks on my study door. He says he hopes I don't mind, but he has mentioned my situation to his own GP, and he – Dr Murray – was wondering if I'd like him to drop in at the flat; just on an informal basis, perhaps to have a cup of tea? I immediately say yes.

Dr Murray has a gentle voice. He says my sponge cake is delicious, and he strokes Tessa behind her ears, which she loves. Harry hasn't been able to take her out for a walk for weeks now.

Later, outside the front door, Dr Murray tells me that he can't tell me what to do as we are not his patients, but, as he puts it, 'I can tell you what I'd do if I were you.' He says he would go directly to the rheumatologist's secretary and describe the level of pain Harry has been suffering since he was discharged, and ask for another appointment.

To my surprise, it works. Harry is given another appointment, and an ambulance is arranged to take him there. This time I'm going to be prepared. 'Dear Dr Wentworth,' I type…

> *Since Harry left hospital at the end of March, his pain has gone on increasing in severity. He is getting weaker and weaker and I think he's lost weight. His appetite is extremely poor. He says that everything tastes awful. He used to love a cup of tea but these days he only drinks water or fizzy lemonade.*
> *Yours sincerely,*
> *Lucy Ansel (Mrs)*

I hope this will convince him that I'm not being hysterical, and that I'm not the cause of what's wrong with Harry. I slip the letter into my bag and go out to get the taxi that Sarah, the department secretary, has kindly ordered for me.

When I reach Harry's bedside he grasps my hand tightly. 'Oh, darling, thank you, thank you so much for coming.'

The curtain is drawn back and someone comes in.

'Are you Dr Wentworth?' I ask, trying to keep my voice steady.

'Yes, and who are you?' Cool, but not dismissive.

'I'm Mr Ansel's wife. Please will you read this letter before examining my husband?'

I hear him take the letter from the envelope. After a brief pause he says, 'Hmm. Yes, you do appear to have lost weight since

I last saw you, Mr Ansel. I think we need to take you back to Walsgrave and do some more investigating. Is that all right?'

'Whatever you think best, Doctor,' says Harry. He can barely speak above a whisper.

They're listening to us at last, I think.

The next day, it is with great sadness that I get in touch with Darren Carter at the guide dog centre in Leamington. I've been worrying for ages about Tessa not getting enough exercise, and now with Harry in hospital for I don't know how long, I realise I can't delay this any longer.

Now I spend my days on campus, and my evenings sitting next to Harry's hospital bed. Each night I ask what's happened to him that day, and every evening for five weeks he says, 'Tests' or 'X-rays', and one evening, 'They took me to another hospital for a scan today.' After that, nothing for two evenings.

They've either run out of tests or they've found something. Now when I stop by the ward sister's office as I usually do to have a word with her, I am greeted with 'Sister's not on duty' or 'We don't know anything.'

One night I cut the usual mantra short. 'I know the sister's not on duty, but she'd better be tomorrow, or else…' And I don't wait for an answer.

When I arrive on the ward the following evening, the sister calls me into her office and asks me to sit down.

'I don't want to sit down. I just want to know what's going on.'

The door opens and Dr Wentworth comes in. 'I didn't want to tell you,' he begins, 'but I have decided that's not fair on you. Mr Ansel's scan has revealed extensive secondary cancers. I'm afraid he is terminally ill. Nothing…nothing can be done.' After a brief pause he goes on, 'We will be sending Mr Ansel home soon. Well, as soon as Sister hears from social services that they have put a support network in place.'

I feel as if I have been turned to stone.

The next morning I knock on Dr Fleming's door.

'Come in,' calls Dr Fleming, and when I enter, 'The chair's in the usual place.'

I sit down. 'They told me last night that Harry's riddled with cancer. He's terminally ill, and nothing can be done.'

'Oh, Lucy. I am so sorry.'

'Can you tell the others? I don't want to have to keep repeating the news.' I stand up. 'I'd better go and get on with my work now.'

A few days later, when I'm dropped off at home and am hurrying up the path to the front door, a voice calls out, 'Mrs Ansel?'

I stop. 'Yes?'

'It's Jane Tranter here. I'm a social worker.'

A social worker! My hackles rise.

'And my colleague Mrs Wallace.'

What do they want?

'May we come in, Mrs Ansel?'

I don't like to be rude. But I don't want these women in my home with me. They have power, and I don't want to talk to them without Harry's supportive presence. I think quickly, and tell them that I'm sorry but it's not convenient, as I am about to be picked up to go to visit my husband in hospital.

'That's exactly why we're here,' says Jane Tranter smoothly. 'We'd like to discuss your husband's care package. We are going to arrange for him to be discharged directly to the hospice in Leamington. You can return to live with your parents, which will be much closer than here for visiting him. And then obviously you'll stay on with them afterwards – you won't be able to live here on your own.'

'What? How dare you?!' Fortunately, I'm already holding the front door key, and I am able to open the door and get inside. A memory of Charlotte Briggs and my mum planning my future together flashes inside my head, and all the old anger and pain surge up inside me. Harry doesn't yet know that he is dying, and already these harpies are trying to muscle in. But Tim will be here soon to pick me up, so I must calm down. I have to be strong for Harry.

11

Term is almost over. The exam results are yet to be announced, and I am slowly packing up my mountain of books, ready to be returned to the RNIB library. I can't make any plans for next year. Apart from anything, life has been so stressful that I think I'll be lucky if I scrape a third.

Harry is discharged from hospital the day before the results come out. I still haven't yet told him what Dr Wentworth told me, but I have spoken to our GP's surgery, and the district nurse will be round soon to see how we are managing. I need to go onto the campus to get my results, but I daren't leave Harry alone in the flat. What if those social workers turn up and blag their way in? I shudder at the thought. I call Tim: he's able to be here in the morning, and Shirley Dyson, my former piano teacher and now a good friend to both me and Harry, can come over at lunchtime. I make sure Harry's settled comfortably in bed and then I head off.

As I pack up the last few bits and pieces in my study, I reflect on how happy I've been in this room for the past two years. I am going to miss it. Then there's a commotion outside: chattering voices and nervous laughter. I go out into the corridor and follow the noise down towards the office, from where Katy materialises and grabs my hand.

'He's coming,' she calls out, 'and he's got a piece of paper in his hand.'

The crowd parts to let Dr Stone through, and then we all surge into the office after him.

'Please,' says Sarah, 'put Lucy out of her misery. Tell her what she's got.'

'Lucy? She's got a 2:1.'

'2:1? Are you sure? That can't be right.'

'What do you mean?'

'I… I was only expecting to get a third.'

'That was never going to happen,' says Dr Fleming, who has just arrived. 'Well, folks,' she adds, 'how about coming over to the bar for a celebratory drink? You too, Lucy – you've earned it.'

'But I ought to go home. Harry will be getting anxious.'

'One drink won't make a difference, then I'll drive you home.'

'Why don't you ring him first?' says Sarah, who's always so sensible. 'Here.' And she hands me the phone.

'Harry, I've got a 2:1!' I gasp when I get him on the phone. 'I can't believe it. It's much, much better than I ever expected.'

'Brilliant! Well done, darling, well done.'

'I'm just going for a drink to celebrate, then Dr Fleming has offered to drive me home. I won't be long.'

When I get home, Shirley is waiting for me by the front door. 'I've been looking out for you. There's something I need to tell you before you go in.'

'Harry's not worse?'

'No, not that. As I got here this afternoon, a car drew up and two sour-faced women got out. When they realised I was coming here, they said I needn't stay and they'd sit with Harry until you came home. They said, "We're going to tell Mr Ansel he's terminally ill and persuade him to go to a hospice, and persuade

Mrs Ansel to return to her parents' home. It's nearer the hospice for visiting." I didn't think you'd like that, so I insisted on staying. Eventually they left.'

'Did they tell him?'

'No, I don't think they liked to with me there.'

I am so relieved. 'Thank you,' I say. 'Thank you!'

Now the district nurse comes every afternoon. Her name is Betty and she is competent and cheerful. She helps Harry back to bed and settles him for the night. I still haven't yet told him that he is dying of cancer. I desperately want to put it off until after my graduation ceremony. I know how much he's looking forward to that, and I really don't want to blight it for him. But it is all so difficult, so awkward: it's not right that I and other people should know, while Harry himself remains ignorant of his diagnosis. But I don't feel strong enough to tell him.

I'd like to ring Father Damian (as Father Hollywell has asked me to call him) to ask for his help and advice, but it's only when I discover that Harry can't hear me on the phone when he's in the bathroom that I'm able to do so. At once Father Damian suggests that he come over for a cup of tea, and I ask him if he'd be able to bring the black skirt that Sarah has made me for graduation. He comes, we discuss arrangements for the graduation ceremony, and Harry and I accept his offer to drive us to the cathedral, where the ceremony is taking place.

'Good,' says Father Damian, rising from his chair. 'I'm glad that's settled. Oh, I almost forgot: I've got your skirt in the car, Lucy. Sarah asked me to bring it over.'

'I'll come out and fetch it,' I say, and then assure Harry, 'I'll be back in a minute, my love.'

In the hall, Father Damian asks, 'What's going on? How can I help you?'

I tell him that I don't know whether, or how, to tell Harry about his diagnosis, and that social services are really worrying me. 'In fact, they're being a nuisance. They keep on turning up, and as well as threatening to tell Harry that he's dying, they're saying I won't be allowed to stay here when he does die. I'm so frightened of them interfering that I daren't go out, in case they come while I'm not here.'

'Just write and tell them that you've got lots of support and you don't want them to visit any more. They'll have to stay away then.'

'Is it that easy to get rid of them?'

'It should be.'

'And what about telling Harry?'

'In my experience, in this situation people sort of divide up into two types: the first lot think you've got it wrong and won't believe you, but the others accept it. I think it's best to tell him. It would be better coming from you, but if you can't do it, I'll do it for you.'

'No,' I say. 'He's my husband, and I love him. It's my responsibility. Thank you, Father.'

12

Friday 13 July 1979. As we're helping Harry out of the bath, Nurse Betty says, 'I'll be along early tomorrow to give you a hand to get ready. You've lost weight, so we'll need to do a tuck-and-pin job to ensure you're smart.'

'Yes, I'm wearing my wedding suit.' After a brief pause, Harry says, 'I expect I'll start putting weight on again soon.'

Ignoring that last remark, Betty says, 'I've also managed to borrow a wheelchair for you.'

'A wheelchair?'

'Please, my love,' I say urgently. 'I know you don't fancy riding in one, but just this once? It's a while since you've been out, and it's a long way to the front of the cathedral.' I pause. 'I can't turn up if you're not going to be there.'

'All right, all right, I'll use it.'

'Thank you. Thank you, darling.'

'Father Damian's taking us, isn't he?'

'Yes, he said he'd come at a quarter past nine. We have to be settled in our seats by ten. Sarah's fetching Mum and Dad, as two wheelchairs won't fit in Father Damian's car.'

'Lucy, you know I'm really, really proud of you, don't you?' Harry asks me the following morning.

'My darling.' I put my arms around him and kiss him. 'I couldn't have done it without you.'

'I didn't do much.'

'Oh, but you did. Masses of practical things, but also putting up with my readers, and with hours of stuff you weren't really interested in. Most of all, being here and loving me.'

'I admit some of the logic went straight past me,' he says, laughing.

There is a ring on the doorbell. 'My, don't you two look smart?' says Father Damian. And then, to Harry, 'Give me your arm, sir: your carriage awaits.'

'Here we are,' says Father Damian as we take our seats in the cathedral. 'Your father's wheelchair is on your right, Lucy, and your mother's sitting to the other side of him.'

'Lucy, you look so distinguished in your cap and cloak,' says Dad.

'It's called a gown, Dad.'

'Well, it suits you.'

'I like the colour of the lining,' says Mum.

I tell her that it's called cerise, which I think is French for 'cherry'. I sit down and take Harry's hand. 'OK, my darling?'

'Yes,' he whispers, lifting my hand to his lips. 'And so proud of my lovely Lucy.'

A soft drift of organ music; footsteps; the rustle of clothes; and the low murmur of voices as dignitaries, academics, students and proud relatives settle into seats all around the cathedral. The voices ebb to a hush as the music swells and the ceremony begins.

Afterwards, I remember little. First, three honorary degrees are awarded; then lists of names are read out as each group of graduands files onto the stage and retreats amid a scatter of applause. At last come the names I know: Kathryn, Marguerite, Marianna, Roger, Anthony, Trevor. Then, 'Lucy Ansel.'

My heart is pounding. The walk to the front goes on forever.

Descending the steps to meet me, the chancellor, Lord Scarman, shakes my hand. 'A wonderful achievement. Very, very well done.'

It is over, and a storm of applause breaks around me. Very, very well done, echoes in my mind. At last I'm back in my seat, and Harry is kissing me.

The rest of the ceremony drifts around me in a rosy haze. Soon everyone is standing and singing, '*God save our gracious Queen…*'

As I emerge into the sunshine it feels as though I am stepping into a different world; one in which angry surf crashes against a solitary rock. No, not now. That can wait.

We have crossed the surf and reached the island that is our quiet, peaceful haven. I have settled Harry in his armchair, and gone to fetch his morphine tablets and a glass of water. As I slowly fill the glass I am silently screaming, No, no, no!

Back in the sitting room, I sit on the arm of Harry's chair. He slides his arm around my waist and rests his head on my shoulder. I turn and kiss the top of his head, and then tentatively ask, 'When…when you were in hospital, my love, what did you think about the tests you had?'

'Not much: in the end, the technicians just seemed to be practising. But it doesn't matter now because I'm sure that soon I'm going to start feeling better.'

My heart misses a beat. 'No, my darling. No, it's not like that.'

I can feel him tensing up. Perhaps he knows what I'm going to say.

'I have to tell you this, because I know it, and I think you should know it too. You're not going to get better. The terrible pain you have…it's not going to get better. Because it's cancer. And it's spread so far that there is nothing they can do.' I am crying now; tears dripping down my face and onto his hair. 'I'm sorry. I'm so, so sorry.'

Harry is silent. I feel as if I can't breathe.

'Harry?' I gasp. 'My darling?'

'That's that, then.' He gives an odd, strangulated laugh. His arm is still around my waist.

Now I start to shake and shudder. I am sobbing; each breath harsh and ragged.

At last he says, 'My darling Lucy. I am so sorry.'

13

It's strange, the calm and the peacefulness that has settled around us now that hope has gone. I no longer try to threaten, coax or cajole Harry into eating. If all he wants is a small handful of dry Sugar Puffs to chew on, that's what I give him, washed down with a glass of fizzy lemonade. When people call round, my heart is no longer in my mouth, afraid every second that they'll say the wrong thing. Now, they can't tell him anything that he doesn't already know.

I find practical solutions to the difficulties that arise, such as dealing with the stuff Harry has to take each day to try to keep his bowels open. I have to be quick as a flash with it or the powder turns to concrete in the glass.

The ritual begins with my asking, 'Ready for the mixture, my love?'

'Yes.'

I put a half-full glass of water into Harry's hand, take a deep breath, open the sachet, tip the foul-smelling powder into the water, and stir. Then a gulp, and it's gone.

Another problem is Harry's medication: the morphine that he has been prescribed for the pain. The GP will prescribe only two days' supply at a time, and the pharmacy is a bus journey away. It is a weary journey that I have to make every other day. I ask the GP if I could have a prescription for a week's worth, and am shocked and upset by his brusque refusal.

'Absolutely not,' he says. 'What if you and your husband made a suicide pact?'

I can hardly believe my ears.

A few days later I am feeling just too exhausted to make the trip to the pharmacy, and burst into tears as I say this to Betty as she is leaving the flat.

'Leave it with me,' she says.

She is as good as her word. I am allowed to name two individuals who can pick up the morphine for me, and Tim and Shirley say they are only too happy to take it in turns.

People start to make farewell visits. Jean and Tony, Bert Edwards, Jill and Dan, Bill and Renée, and Harry's brothers Arnold and Peter. In early August, Harry's sister Lily comes for the day. It feels good to show her our happy home. We always intended to have her to stay once my exams were over, but now it is too late.

I go out to the chippy to get fish and chips for dinner. As I come out, clutching the warm paper bag to my chest, I am hailed by Mr Khan, who has come out of his own shop to speak to me.

'Mrs Ansel,' he calls out. 'I haven't seen Mr Ansel for a while.'

'No, he's very ill. Well, actually he's dying.'

'I am so sorry. Please may I give you a lift home in my van?'

'I was just coming to your shop to get some lemonade. We've run out, and it's the only thing Harry drinks now.'

'Let me get it.' Then he helps me into his van.

When we pull up outside the flat, he places a slip of paper in my hand.

'This is my number. You need anything, any time, day, night, just ring, and I come.'

My eyes fill with tears. 'That's so, so kind.'

'Please,' says Mr Khan. 'Let me be your son.'

As Lily and I eat our fish and chips, and Harry toys with a couple of chips, Lily says innocently, 'I love the way there's so much going on here. I can see the people in the house opposite, and it's lovely watching the passers-by. There's only a brick wall to look at outside my living-room window.'

That night in bed, I tell Harry that it has never occurred to me that we are on display like that. If Lily could see the people opposite, they must be able to see us. 'I'll remember to shut the kitchen door in future,' I say.

'Well,' says Harry, 'I don't mind them seeing us being happy.'

I put an arm across his chest. 'We were so lucky to find each other.'

Some visitors are awkward, as though Harry's approaching death holds up a mirror to their own mortality; a fact too uncomfortable for them to contemplate. They smile brightly and tell him he'll be up and about in no time. Sometimes he's fierce in reply: 'No, I won't. I'm dying.' Then they hastily take their leave.

My old friend Janet is weird in a different way. She rings up and tells Harry that she can't come and see him because it would upset her too much. 'That's fine,' says Harry. Later he tells me that Janet pretended she could hear her doorbell ringing, as an excuse to end the conversation.

Once a week my sister Rosemary comes over from Leamington. She reads the local paper to Harry, and chats with him about the stories. He is relaxed with her; calm. She wishes she could do more, but I am very grateful for what she does.

Julie, my bridesmaid, who moved to London soon after Harry and I got married, takes time off work and comes to see us. The three of us spend a happy afternoon reminiscing, and I recall when Harry and I went to see Julie in London soon after the wedding: 'I don't think I ever told you, Harry, that that was the very first time I'd been on an escalator. My heart sank when you said, "You don't mind escalators, darling, do you?"'

'You never said.'

'No. I just decided to trust you.'

'You did very well,' says Harry. 'Excellent for a novice. I never even guessed.'

I rarely leave the flat now. We have a home help, called Margaret, who comes most mornings to clean and shop for us. Nurse Betty continues to come every afternoon. Mr Khan drops off extra groceries. Friends and family come and go.

On Sundays, however, I still go out to church. A group of parishioners take it in turns to give me a lift there and back. I draw great comfort from the hymns. 'Guide Me, O Thou Great Redeemer': I know myself as a pilgrim in a barren land. When the congregation sings 'Lead Us, Heavenly Father, Lead Us', I am transported back to our wedding day; walking up the aisle on Dad's arm towards Harry as he waited for me before the altar: *'Guard us, guide us, keep us, feed us, For we have no help but Thee.'* And most comforting of all, 'Be Still, My Soul':

> *Be still, my soul; the Lord is on thy side;*
> *Bear patiently the cross of grief or pain.*
> *Leave to thy God to order and provide;*
> *In every change He faithful will remain.*

Joining in the refrain, I pray, Help me to trust You, Lord.

14

Feet are always tramping in and out of our small flat; relentlessly wearing away, it seems to me, the little time Harry and I have left together.

Betty comes just after half past three each day. 'Hello, Harry, how are you feeling today?'

'A bit tired, but not too bad' is his usual refrain.

It's me who tells her about his restless nights and occasional bouts of weeping, when he lets the pain build up too much before asking for morphine. In time I get to recognise the early signs: agitated movements in his chair, or a restless murmuring in his sleep as he tries to ease the increasing discomfort, which, if ignored for long, topples over the edge into raging, gnawing pain. In the end I say, 'You need the pills, yes?', and he squeezes my hand in reply. As Shirley and Tim bring Harry's morphine, their visits are always welcome. I am grateful to them, but I also experience them as further sets of feet invading our precious space and time.

July slides by. Each day, when everyone has gone, we listen to our favourite radio programmes or put some music on the record player, while I sit on the arm of Harry's chair or beside the bed: close together, always holding hands, clinging to each other as though we can slow down the passage of time. On good days, we play Scrabble.

'Your turn to start, darling.'

'I've got fourteen for "day". Double word.'

'Mm… I'm turning it into "holiday". That's four, double letter plus five, six, seven…fourteen.'

By the second week in August, Harry can no longer walk the few steps from the bed to the bathroom or his armchair.

'We'll find a way to manage,' I assure him. 'Do you remember how you used to push me to the loo at Chester Grove when my leg was in plaster? In the end, if I wanted to go anywhere, people would sing out, "Harry'll push her." Well, now it's my turn to do the same for you.'

'But how?'

I have to sound confident about this. I get out Harry's wheelchair and, with the brakes on, we manage to manoeuvre him into it. 'I'm going to walk backwards,' I tell him, 'pulling you towards me. I once told my orthopaedic specialist that I could walk better backwards than forwards. He didn't believe me, so I gave him a demo.'

Harry laughs. 'You're amazing.'

One afternoon, when as usual I hand him his morphine tablets and glass of water, instead of a quiet 'Thank you' there is a coughing, spluttering sound. Harry is struggling to swallow the tablets. Eventually he lies back against my arm, frightened and exhausted.

'Lucy, darling, you won't leave me, will you?'

'Of course not, darling, of course not.' I stroke his head and kiss him, and hold him close.

Later on, when Betty comes out of the bedroom, I beckon her into the kitchen and describe how Harry nearly choked when I gave him his last lot of pills.

'Hmm, that's difficult. If he can't take the morphine by mouth, he'll have to go back to hospital.'

'But neither of us wants that.'

'I don't think you could manage it in liquid form. But there is another way you could try. When is he likely to need the next dose?'

'Around six o'clock.'

'I'll come back then and see if you can manage to crush the tablets.'

Sure enough, Betty reappears at six on the dot. 'Hello, Harry, ready for your tablets yet?'

'Please.'

'I'm going to teach Lucy how to crush them. Good, I see you've got everything ready: a dessert spoon, a teaspoon, a small medicine glass, and a jug of water. First you need the glass three-quarters full. Now take two tablets out of the bottle. Put one of them in the bowl of the dessert spoon, and place the bowl of the teaspoon on top.'

'Like this?' I press a finger on the neck of the teaspoon.

'I think you'd find it easier if you put your two forefingers under the bowl of the bigger spoon. Now try pressing down your left thumb into the bowl of the teaspoon.'

I feel the tablet crunch between the spoons.

'Yes, that's it. Tip the powder into the glass, and now do the second tablet. Give them a good stir. Harry, it won't taste very nice, but see if you can swallow it.'

Harry takes the glass and gulps the mixture down. 'Yuck.'

'Lemonade?' I suggest.

'Please, love.'

'That went better than I hoped,' says Betty. 'I'll ring in the morning to see how you got on during the night.'

As I let her out, I tell her again that neither Harry nor I wants him to be admitted to hospital.

I become so adept at crushing the pills that I can get out of bed in the middle of the night and, within two or three minutes, grind the tablets between the spoons and mix the powder in the medicine glass. Once Harry has gulped down the dose, I am ready with some lemonade. In no time at all I'm back in bed, snuggling up to him, and within ten or fifteen minutes we are both asleep once more.

One morning the postman comes with a load of hefty canvas bags, which he hands over to Margaret and which she lugs into the living room, exclaiming at their weight.

'That'll be Lucy's law books,' says Harry. 'She's starting a course at the poly in the last week in September.'

'Where shall I put them?'

'On the table under the window for now,' I tell her. 'I'll sort them out later.'

'Goodness, I'd have thought you'd have had enough of studying,' says Margaret.

'It's an addiction,' says Harry, 'but it keeps her out of mischief.'

I laugh and switch on the radio.

One afternoon as Harry is dozing in his armchair, I fetch a book from the shelf and begin to read, turning the pages with great care so as not to disturb his sleep.

Waking, he says, 'I wonder what the weather's doing?'

I carry on reading.

'Do you think it's going to rain?'

I snap at him. 'I'm trying to read.'

'Sorry,' he murmurs.

'No, *I'm* sorry.' I shut the book and sit down on the arm of his chair. There'll be time enough later to read any number of law books. I slide an arm around his neck and bend down to kiss him. 'It'll be September the day after next. We often have nice, settled weather then.'

On Saturday, I slide out from under the duvet and into my slippers, and walk to the bedroom door. 'Just going to get a cup of tea.' A few minutes later, I drop a gentle kiss on Harry's forehead. 'Would you like some breakfast, love?'

There's no reply, and my heart misses a beat. I run into the living room and grab the phone.

'Betty, Harry's not talking to me. I don't know if he's conscious.'

Betty says she'll be right over, and that she'll alert the doctor too. I go back to the bedroom, sit down on the bed and pick up Harry's hand. His pulse goes *dup, dup, dup*; faint but regular.

'Please hurry, Betty,' I say to myself, and then I hear the doorbell.

'Feeling a bit poorly, are we?' Betty says when she comes in. 'Put the kettle on, Lucy, I'll join you in a minute. Harry, do you want a wee? You can just go now: I've got a bottle in place. There, does that feel better?'

'Mmm.'

Betty tells me that a locum doctor's coming out. She herself can't stay; they are really short-handed. When the locum arrives he spends four or five minutes with Harry, and then tells me that he needs to be in hospital, so he's going to ring for an ambulance. I tell him that if he does, I'll barricade the flat and not let anyone in at all.

'But he must. He could die this weekend, and if he does the undertakers won't remove the body until Monday.'

'That's nothing after everything we've been through. He's not leaving here alive. That's my last word.'

I think the locum realises that he has come up against an immovable object. He backs down, but says I must promise to get someone to come over to be with me, so that I'm not alone.

I see the doctor out, and go back to Harry's side. 'All right, love, he's gone.'

Harry gives my hand a feeble squeeze. 'They're not going to take me to hospital, are they?' he whispers.

'No. I said if they tried it, I'd barricade us in. Don't worry, I won't let them. I'm just going to ask Shirley to come over, just to keep the doctor happy. I'll make up a bed for her on the sofa.'

'Promise me something, my darling.'

'What?' I say warily.

'When I die, you won't go and live with your mother.'

'Oh, Harry!' I give a big smile. 'I promise.'

I leave the room to let Shirley in, but return when Harry rings the little bell I have put beside the bed.

'Lucy,' he whispers. 'Bread-and-butter pudding?'

'Of course, love, I'll make you bread-and-butter pudding, but it'll take an hour to cook. Would you like something else in the meantime?'

'Banana,' he whispers.

Nothing but dry Sugar Puffs for weeks, and now bread-and-butter pudding and a banana. I pick a banana out of the fruit bowl and return to the bedroom. Sitting on the edge of the bed, I break off a morsel and slide it into his mouth.

'More,' he murmurs, and another morsel follows the first.

Then I construct a bread-and-butter pudding and put it in the oven. 'I don't suppose he'll eat much of this, if any,' I tell Shirley, 'but we can finish it.'

Harry's bell rings again. I tell him that the pudding's in the oven.

'I want Father Damian,' he whispers. 'Please, Lucy, I want Father Damian.'

Father Damian, I know, is in Wales today, but he's due back in the morning to take Mass. I tell Harry that, and he nods.

On Sunday, Harry wants more banana. I pinch off little bits and slide them into his mouth. I can feel the sun caressing my hair, and a dark rage rises in me. How dare the sun shine when Harry's slipping away from me? How dare it peer in here?

Then Father Damian is beside me, taking the banana from my hand. I give him the bedside seat, and move to the ottoman opposite the end of the bed. A great sense of peace fills the room.

'Is my wife here?'

'She's sitting in the sunshine by the window,' says Father Damian.

'Ah,' Harry murmurs. 'I need to have her near.'

'Of course,' says Father Damian. 'That's as it should be.'

For the rest of the afternoon, Harry drifts in and out of sleep.

Father Damian has left, and Shirley, who's spending the night again, won't be here for another couple of hours. Once again, the room is in shadow.

'Lucy?'

'Yes, darling?'

'Music.'

'What would you like?'

'Our tune,' Harry breathes.

I slip into the living room and come back with a cassette tape, which I slide into the machine. Beethoven's Piano Concerto No. 1 fills the room, and at once I am back in the principal's office in Chester Grove in 1973, sitting on the desk with Harry's arm around me as we listen to John Lill playing at the Proms. The slow music flows around the room.

Then it stops, and Harry whispers, 'Again.'

Three times I rewind the tape. Three times those haunting notes cascade over us.

At seven o'clock the next morning, I slowly withdraw my hand from Harry's and slide out from under the duvet. I walk round to his side of the bed and listen. *Ssshh…* A pause. *Ssshhh*, comes his shallow breath. Bending, I stroke his head and drop a gentle kiss on his mouth before gliding to the kitchen and switching on the kettle. I pour two cups of tea, and take them into the living room.

'Shirley,' I whisper. 'Tea?'

We drink in silence; then I put down my cup and go back into the bedroom. I step into a profound stillness. Harry has gone.

Father Damian takes everything in hand, accompanying me to collect the death certificate, to visit the registrar, and to arrange matters with the undertakers. I haven't been outside the flat for ten days, and it is a surprise to find that the ordinary world is still here, though today it appears to be weeping; a soft mizzle that mingles with my tears.

Later – much later – I am expecting Shirley, who is coming back to spend the night with me. I hear the doorbell and go to open the door.

'It's me, darling.' Mum steps forwards and holds me tight. 'Let's get your case, and we can be going home. Jill and Dan are waiting in the car.'

It would be good to be spoiled for a while: not to have to think about anything, or have meals to cook or washing-up to do. But then I am back sitting on the side of the bed, holding Harry's hand and making him a promise.

'Lucy,' says Mum sharply. 'You're not listening to me.'

'Yes, Mum. No, no – I mean, no: I'm staying here.'

'But you can't stay here alone.'

The social worker's voice echoes in my mind: You won't be allowed to stay here once Mr Ansel dies.

'Please, Lucy,' Mum cajoles. 'I promised your dad I'd bring you back with me.'

'No, Mum. I've told you before: this is my home now.'

The doorbell rings again.

'I'll get it,' says Mum.

'No,' I say firmly. '*I'll* get it.' I open the door. 'Come in, Shirley. I've put the kettle on for tea. Mum, you'll have a cup before you go?'

Epilogue

As I was picking some raspberries just now – the nets are a fearful struggle but, oh, it is worth it for the taste of the sun-warmed berries in your mouth – the smell of the earth triggered such a sharp memory of my dad when I was little; when he was a farm labourer and his clothes always gave off a faint smell of earth and hay. And cow, too. I smile at the thought of a cow transplanted into my little inner-city back garden. I remember how I used to go out into the lane on my tricycle to meet Dad when he got back from work, and how he'd pretend to race me home, wobbling slowly behind me on his bike so that I could reach the gate first. It was Dad who had lifted me onto Stephen's new tricycle when I was four, saying, 'Oh, let her have a go.' It was Dad who set me going with his belief in me.

Dad died the year after I lost Harry. And the year after that, in 1981, David Scott Blackhall died. One, two, three. It was a dark time, with each death throwing me back to the one that had gone before. I had been listening to *In Touch* the week before David died, without knowing, of course, that it would be his final episode. He was the first person I ever heard talk publicly about the experience of going blind. I was thirteen then, and I had been blind for four years. David sounded much older than me, and hadn't gone blind until he was in his forties, but when I heard him describe the fear, the panic, and the belief that this couldn't possibly last forever, it was as if he was there inside my head, talking directly to me. Nobody who is not blind can imagine the terror of realising that you are never going to see again; that you will live in darkness for the rest of your life. David made me feel for the first time that I wasn't completely alone, and in the years that followed I drew comfort from the warmth of his voice on the radio, his humour, and his understanding. Then on one of his programmes he had a guest from America to talk about the long cane, and when I heard about that, my life changed dramatically. I was too small and frail to be able to benefit from a guide dog, but the long cane gave me mobility and independence.

And it gave me Harry. In a sort of roundabout way, David was instrumental in bringing us together, and then when I discovered that he and Harry actually knew, liked and respected each other, it seemed to me that David had taken on the role of a fairy godfather, bestowing a blessing on our marriage. Harry and David were the same age. In the end, I didn't get the full ten years with Harry that we had joked about before we were married. But the years I did have with him were so happy and exciting, so filled with love, that the grief I felt at losing him was mitigated by a constant thankfulness that I had ever found him, and that I had had those precious years with him before he became ill.

When I was a small child, my parents were told that there were two things I would never do: I would not survive into adulthood, and if somehow, miraculously, I did survive, I would never find love. My rebellion against those judgements has shaped my life. Over and over I have met with low expectations, which over and over I have defied.

Things were hard when Harry died. I was so lonely; lonelier than I had ever been before. But he had made me strong. I stayed in our flat, and I did my law course at the polytechnic. It was difficult to find work afterwards, though, and I was feeling depressed (and struggling to hide that from my family) when one day I bumped into Monica, my old champion from the careers office at Warwick University, and heard from her about a project in Nottingham that was looking for someone to collect data on disabled graduates and what they'd done since getting their degrees. The pay was minimal – less than what I was getting on benefits – but it was a foot in the door of employment, and it meant that I myself was no longer adding to the statistics of unemployed disabled graduates. From there I got a job as a disability equality officer with the city council, and when, a couple of years later, I saw a job with a much wider remit being advertised by Bristol City Council, I barely hesitated before applying for it; only long enough to conjure up Harry's voice in my head: This is your career, Lucy. Of course you must move to Bristol. Yes, this is my career. I didn't make it to the Houses of Parliament as I once dreamed, but I've done other things for people with disabilities. I have discovered that I'm good at detail, that I'm good at identifying practical solutions to problems, and that I'm good at motivating people. I've been here in Bristol for more than a quarter of a century now – sometimes I can hardly believe that – and this is my home; this is where I belong.

Rosemary visits two or three times a year. I am utterly ruthless when she comes: I have her out in the garden, digging, planting or weeding, depending on the season. Mum used to come, too. We made our peace before she died. She fought against it, but in the end she let me live my own life. She loved me, I know. When my brother Stephen was in his forties he lost his job, but he put himself through a degree in computing and IT, and now he has a very well-paid job in Manchester. He remarried after his divorce and has two stepchildren. I see them at least once a year. Rosemary's Simon came to university here, then went away, came back and got married, and I now have a grand-niece and a grand-nephew who live only ten minutes away from me. I am awfully fond of Simon and his family.

Some years ago my hearing (or what hearing I had left) began to deteriorate rapidly. Modern hearing aids are amazing. I can hardly believe it when I think back to my first hearing aid, the one I got at Brilbeck House, and how it was like having to cart around a huge piece of luggage. So much has changed since those days: for writing I use a Braille laptop that speaks back to me, and my wheelchair is easily manoeuvrable (comparatively speaking) and under my control. But even with my direction-sensitive hearing aid I was struggling to hear during large meetings, and also in one-to-one situations if there was a lot of background noise. During my years with the council I had become a regular convenor of small meetings in Park Street's many tea and coffee shops; I've always believed that tea and biscuits are a great help to decision-making. But the background noise became too much for me.

I worried about giving up my job, and losing my colleagues and friends. But I got freelance work as a disability consultant, made new contacts and new friends, and not having a full-time job means I can spend more time on my old passions and my new ones. My old passions are playing the piano and reading. My new passions are gardening and writing. My small garden is designed for a wheelchair user: it has a smooth, wide path running between raised beds where I grow plants and flowers for their smell, for the bees, and, yes, for the deliciousness of the raspberries (dratted nets notwithstanding). Clumps of lavender and rosemary grow out from the raised borders, so that they brush against my wheelchair as I pass and release their scent into the air.

And as for writing, well, about ten years ago a disabled poet friend begged and pleaded with me to go to a workshop he had been given funding to run. He was worried that no one was going to turn up and he'd just have to sit there on his own. Well, a handful of people did turn up, and it was a wonderful three hours, and the workshop morphed into a poetry group that meets once a month, and I've been writing poetry compulsively ever since. At about the same time as I discovered poetry, I attended a day school, put on by the access unit at Bristol University and run by a local writer, on writing memoir, family history, and autobiography, and it gave me so many ideas I began to get scared that I wasn't going to live long enough to explore them all. But here I am, still working away on them and trying to wrestle them into shape and language.

Harry knew that, for all my tears and all my fears, deep down I am truly tenacious. In the end, you must not let anyone or anything divert you from what you want to do and who you want to be. In the end, as Harry knew I would, I bought the red coat.

Printed in Great Britain
by Amazon